OXFORD MEDICAL PUBLICATIONS

Emergencies in Respiratory Medicine

**Published and forthcoming titles in the Emergencies in...
series:**

Emergencies in Anaesthesia
Edited by Keith Allman, Andrew McIndoe, and Iain H. Wilson

Emergencies in Cardiology
Edited by Saul G. Myerson, Robin P. Choudhury, and Andrew Mitchell

Emergencies in Clinical Surgery
Edited by Chris Callaghan, Chris Watson and Andrew Bradley

Emergencies in Critical Care
Edited by Martin Beed, Richard Sherman, and Ravi Mahajan

Emergencies in Nursing
Edited by Philip Downing

Emergencies in Obstetrics and Gynaecology
Edited by S. Arulkumaran

Emergencies in Oncology
Edited by Martin Scott-Brown, Roy A.J. Spence, and Patrick G. Johnston

Emergencies in Paediatrics and Neonatology
Edited by Stuart Crisp and Jo Rainbow

Emergencies in Palliative and Supportive Care
Edited by David Currow and Katherine Clark

Emergencies in Primary Care
Chantal Simon, Karen O'Reilly, John Buckmaster, and Robin Proctor

Emergencies in Psychiatry
Basant Puri and Ian Treasaden

Emergencies in Radiology
Edited by Richard Graham and Ferdia Gallagher

Emergencies in Respiratory Medicine
Edited by Robert Parker, Catherine Thomas, and Lesley Bennett

Head, Neck and Dental Emergencies
Edited by Mike Perry

Medical Emergencies in Dentistry
Nigel Robb and Jason Leitch

Emergencies in Respiratory Medicine

Edited by

Robert Parker
Specialist Registrar
General and Respiratory Medicine
Oxford, UK

Catherine Thomas
Specialist Registrar
General and Respiratory Medicine
Oxford, UK

Lesley Bennett
Consultant Respiratory Physician
Oxford Centre for Respiratory Medicine
Churchill Hospital
Oxford, UK

OXFORD
UNIVERSITY PRESS

OXFORD

UNIVERSITY PRESS

Great Clarendon Street, Oxford OX2 6DP

Oxford University Press is a department of the University of Oxford.
It furthers the University's objective of excellence in research, scholarship,
and education by publishing worldwide in

Oxford New York

Auckland Cape Town Dar es Salaam Hong Kong Karachi
Kuala Lumpur Madrid Melbourne Mexico City Nairobi
New Delhi Shanghai Taipei Toronto

With offices in

Argentina Austria Brazil Chile Czech Republic France Greece
Guatemala Hungary Italy Japan Poland Portugal Singapore
South Korea Switzerland Thailand Turkey Ukraine Vietnam

Oxford is a registered trade mark of Oxford University Press
in the UK and in certain other countries

Published in the United States
by Oxford University Press Inc., New York

© Oxford University Press, 2007

The moral rights of the authors have been asserted
Database right Oxford University Press (maker)

First published 2007

British Library Cataloguing in Publication Data

Data available

Library of Congress Cataloging in Publication Data

Data available

Typeset by Newgen Imaging Systems (P) Ltd., Chennai, India
Printed in Italy
on acid-free paper by
Legoprint S.p.A.

ISBN 978-0-19-920244-7

10 9 8 7 6 5 4 3 2 1

Preface

Respiratory medicine encompasses a substantial part of all emergencies a doctor or other healthcare professional will encounter and provides a large workload for those involved in acute medical care. *Emergencies in Respiratory Medicine* is part of a series from Oxford University Press intended to meet the need for practical advice in these situations.

The book has been coordinated by a consultant and two specialist registrars in respiratory medicine. It was written by specialist registrars in general medicine, respiratory medicine, intensive care medicine, anaesthesia and radiology plus a specialist in respiratory physiotherapy. It aims to provide front-line healthcare professionals with the information and skills to manage acute respiratory emergencies, and also provide background knowledge to deal with acute conditions in those with known chronic respiratory disease.

It is divided into five sections. The first covers common acute respiratory presentations, and the second moves onto more specific acute clinical scenarios. The third section provides more didactic information on a variety of acute respiratory conditions and relevant features of some chronic respiratory diseases on which a general physician may be asked to provide on-call advice. The last two sections cover practical issues and investigations.

It is impossible for this book to be exhaustive, and it was not conceived as such. It is intended that it should be used in conjunction with others, in particular its sister publication the *Oxford Handbook of Respiratory Medicine*.

Contents

Part 5: Practical and management issues

Part 6: Investigations

Contributors

Matt Brookes
Specialist Registrar
Radiology
London, UK

Ali Gates
Respiratory Physiotherapist
Department of Physiotherapy
Churchill Hospital
Oxford, UK

James Hull
Specialist Registrar
General and Respiratory Medicine
London, UK

Christopher Loew
Specialist Registrar
Anaesthesia and Intensive Care
Medicine
Oxford, UK

Robert MacKenzie Ross
Specialist Registrar
General and Respiratory Medicine
Oxford, UK

Robert Parker
Specialist Registrar
General and Respiratory Medicine
Oxford, UK

Anjani Prasad
Consultant Physician
Buckinghamshire Hospitals
NHS Trust
Aylesbury, UK

Najib Rahman
Specialist Registrar and Pleural
Research Fellow
General and Respiratory
Medicine
Oxford, UK

Fran Sinfield
Senior Respiratory
Physiotherapist
Department of Physiotherapy
Churchill Hospital
Oxford, UK

Andrew Stanton
Specialist Registrar
General and Respiratory
Medicine
Oxford, UK

Catherine Thomas
Specialist Registrar
General and Respiratory Medicine
Oxford, UK

Sam Waddy
Specialist Registrar
General and Intensive Care
Medicine
Oxford, UK

David Waine
Specialist Registrar and Cystic
Fibrosis Research Fellow
General and Respiratory Medicine
Birmingham, UK

Symbols and abbreviations

A–a	alveolar to arterial gradient
ABG	arterial blood gas
ABPA	allergic bronchopulmonary aspergillosis
ACE	angiotensin-converting enzyme
AFB	acid-fast bacillus
AIDS	acquired immune deficiency syndrome
AIP	acute interstitial pneumonia
ANA	antinuclear antibody
ANCA	antinuclear cytoplasmic antibody
APACHE	Apache Physiology and Chronic Health Evaluation
APTT	activated partial thromboplastin time
ARDS	acute respiratory distress syndrome
ATS	American Thoracic Society
AVM	arteriovenous malformation
BAL	bronchoalveolar lavage
bd	twice a day
BIPAP	bi-level positive airways pressure
BMI	body mass index (kg/metres^2)
BNP	Brain Naturetic Peptide
BTS	British Thoracic Society
CAP	community-acquired pneumonia
CCDC	Consultant for communicable disease control
CCF	congestive cardiac failure
CF	cystic fibrosis
CFA	cryptogenic fibrosing alveolitis
CFTR	Cystic fibrosis transmembrane conductance regulator
CMV	cytomegalovirus
CO	carbon monoxide
COHb	carboxyhaemoglobin
CO_2	carbon dioxide
COP	cryptogenic organizing pneumonia
COPD	chronic obstructive pulmonary disease
CPAP	continuous positive airway pressure
CRP	C-reactive protein

CSF	cerebrospinal fluid
CT	computerized tomography
CTPA	computerized tomographic pulmonary angiogram
CVA	cardiovascular accident
CXR	chest radiograph
DIC	disseminated intravascular coagulation
DIP	desquamative interstitial pneumonitis
DVT	deep vein thrombosis
ECG	electrocardiogram
Echo	echocardiogram
ELISA	enzyme-linked immunosorbent assay
EMG	electromyogram
ENT	ear, nose, and throat
EPAP	expiratory positive airways pressure
ERS	European Respiratory Society
ESR	erythrocyte sedimentation rate
ESS	Epworth sleepiness scale/score
FBC	full blood count
FEV_1	forced expiratory volume in 1 second
FiO_2	fractional inspired oxygen
FNA	fine needle aspirate
FRC	functional residual capacity
FVC	forced vital capacity
g	gram
GBM	glomerular basement membrane
GI	gastrointestinal
GORD	gastro-oesophageal reflux disease
GU	genitourinary
HAART	highly active antiretroviral therapy
HACE	high altitude cerebral oedema
HAP	Hospital acquired pneumonia
HAPE	high altitude pulmonary oedema
Hb	haemoglobin
HCO_3	bicarbonate
HHT	hereditary haemorrhagic telangiectasia
HIV	human immunodeficiency virus
HP	hypersensitivity pneumonitis
HRCT	high resolution computerized tomography
HSV	herpes simplex virus

ICD	intercostal drain
ICU	intensive care unit
IgE	immunoglobulin E
IgG	immunoglobulin G
IgM	immunoglobulin M
IIP	idiopathic interstitial pneumonia
ILD	interstitial lung disease
IM	intramuscular
INR	international normalized ratio
IPAP	inspiratory positive airways pressure
IPF	idiopathic pulmonary fibrosis
ITU	intensive therapy unit
IV	intravenous
IVC	inferior vena cava
JVP	jugular venous pressure
kCO	carbon monoxide transfer factor
L	litre
LAM	lymphangioleiomyomatosis
LDH	lactate dehydrogenase
LFTs	liver function tests
LIP	lymphoid interstitial pneumonia
LMWH	low molecular weight heparin
LTOT	long-term oxygen therapy
MC & S	microscopy, culture, and sensitivity
MDI	metered dose inhaler
MDR-TB	multidrug-resistant TB
MDT	multidisciplinary team
mg	milligrams
MI	myocardial infarction
min	minute
MRI	magnetic resonance imaging
MRSA	methicillin (or multiply) resistant *Staphylococcus aureus*
MSU	mid stream urine
MTB	mycobacterium tuberculosis
MU	megaunits
ng	nanograms
NIPPV	non-invasive positive pressure ventilation
NIV	non-invasive ventilation
NO	nitric oxide

NO_2	nitrogen dioxide
NSAID	non-steroidal anti-inflammatory drug
NSIP	non-specific interstitial pneumonia
NTM	non-tuberculous mycobacteria
OCP	oral contraceptive pill
od	once a day
OSA	obstructive sleep apnoea
$PaCO_2$	arterial carbon dioxide tension
PAH	pulmonary arterial hypertension
PaO_2	arterial oxygen tension
PAP	pulmonary artery pressure
PC20	provocative concentration (of histamine or methacholine) causing a 20% fall in FEV1
PCP	*pneumocystis carinii* (now *jiroveci*) pneumonia
PE	pulmonary embolus
PEEP	positive end expiratory pressure
PEFR	peak expiratory flow rate
PEG	percutaneous endoscopic gastrostomy
PFTs	pulmonary function test
PHT	pulmonary hypertension
PND	paroxysmal nocturnal dyspnoea
PO	orally/by mouth
PPH	primary pulmonary hypertension
prn	as required
PT	prothrombin time
PTX	pneumothorax
PUD	Peptic Ulcer Disease
qds	four times a day
RAST	radioallergosorbent test
RBBB	right bundle branch block
RB-ILD	respiratory bronchiolitis-associated interstitial lung disease
RCP	Royal College of Physicians
RCT	randomized controlled trial
REM	rapid eye movement sleep
rPTH	parathyroid hormone related peptide
RSV	respiratory syncytial virus
RV	residual volume
RVH	right ventricular hypertrophy
SaO_2	arterial oxygen saturation

SARS	severe acquired respiratory syndrome
SBE	subacute bacterial endocarditis
SE	side-effect
SLE	systemic lupus erythematosus
SIADH	syndrome of inappropriate anti-diuretic hormone secretion
SOB	shortness of breath
SVC	superior vena cava
SVCO	superior vena caval obstruction
TB	tuberculosis
TBB	transbronchial biopsy
tds	three times a day
TFT	thyroid function tests
TLC	total lung capacity
TLCO	total lung carbon monoxide transfer factor
TSH	thyroid-stimulating hormone
U & E	urea and electrolytes
UIP	usual interstitial pneumonia
URTI	upper respiratory tract infection
USS	ultrasound scan
V/Q	ventilation/perfusion ratio
VAP	ventilator acquired pneumonia
VATS	video-assisted thoracoscopic surgery
VC	vital capacity
VTE	venous thromboembolism
WBC	white blood cell count
WCC	white cell count
WHO	World Health Organisation
ZN	Ziehl–Neelson
μg	micrograms

Part 1

Presentation

The peri-arrest patient (incorporating BLS and ALS)

☢ Basic life support

Occasionally you will be the first person on the scene. Doctors get used to running arrests, so do not freeze when you walk into a cubicle and find the unresponsive patient – just do the basics.

These algorithms are included as a reminder of previously learnt basic and advanced life support skills as taught on the appropriate resuscitation council courses. For further information and reading: www.resus.org.uk

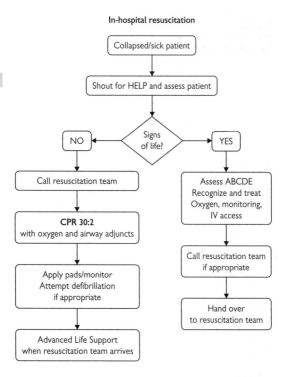

In-hospital resuscitation

Fig. 1.1 Current basic life support guidelines. (With kind permission from the Resuscitation Council.)

☠ Advanced life support

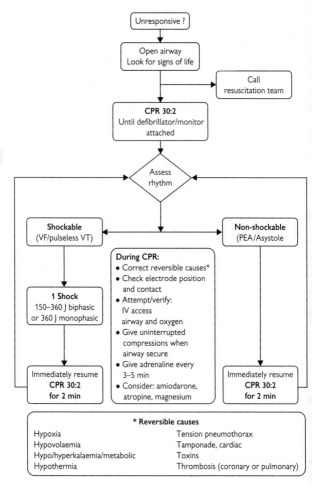

Fig. 1.2 Current advanced life support guidelines. (With kind permission from the resuscitation council.)

:☠: The peri-arrest patient

Junior doctors are frequently paralysed when faced with a nearly but not quite arrested patient. Remember to go back to basics.

The key is simultaneous assessment and treatment.

►► Initial assessment and actions

Nominate a colleague to get IV access, order the CXR, and do the ABGs. While performing the assessment below ask the patient for a focused history if possible; otherwise ask the nurses and/or nominate someone to look through (and read aloud) the recent admission notes and the drug chart.

- Airway – if compromised
  - Perform basic airway manoeuvres (head tilt and chin lift or jaw thrust) and insert an oropharyngeal or nasopharyngeal airway if required and tolerated.
  - Call for anaesthetic help if needed.
- Breathing
  - Apply high-flow oxygen.
  - Respiratory rate.
  - Oxygen saturations.
  - Quick examination for pneumothorax, massive effusion, silent chest, pulmonary oedema.
  - Request portable CXR urgently.
  - ABGs.
- Circulation
  - Heart rate, rhythm.
  - Blood pressure.
  - JVP.
  - Capillary refill time.
  - Quick palpation of the abdomen (distended? pulsatile mass?).
  - Insert large-bore IV cannula and send FBC, U&E, Clotting ± group and save.
  - 12 lead ECG.
  - 250–500 ml fluid bolus unless heart failure/intrinsic cardiogenic shock.
- Disability
  - Capillary blood glucose.
  - AVPU assessment (Alert, responds to Voice, Pain, Unresponsive).
  - Pupils.
  - Neck stiffness.
  - Tone, plantars.

Diagnosis and treatment

The differential diagnosis of a collapsed patient is wide. At this stage you need to decide what the priority treatment is and act. Many patients will have combinations of the causes listed, e.g. a patient recently returned to the ward from intensive care may have critical care neuromyopathy and a hospital-acquired pneumonia, both causing compromise, and then become 'tipped over' by accumulation of opiate analgesia.

Airway compromise
► Call early for anaesthetic help.
● Most commonly due to decreased level of consciousness. Consider:
  • ⚠ **Opiates** (give naloxone 400 mcg IV stat up to 2 mg repeated at
    intervals of 2–3 min to a maximum of 10 mg). Remember that the
    half-life of naloxone is short and that half-time of opiates can be
    very prolonged in the critically ill.
  • **Glucose** (if low give 50 ml 5% glucose IV stat). Diabetic patients
    may be symptomatically hypoglycaemic at higher levels, treat
    if <4.0.
  • **Intracerebral event**: bleed, coning, infection. Urgent CT.
● Primary airway pathology
  • **Anaphylaxis** and **anaphylactoid** reactions (📖 Chapter 18). Give IM
    adrenaline 0.5–1 mg. Hydrocortisone 200 mg IV. Chlorphenamine
    10 mg IV. Adrenaline nebulizer 1 mg/ml can also be used.
  • **Infection**: epiglottitis, diphtheria, uvula infection/inflammation.
● Uncommonly, inhaled foreign body (📖 Chapter 11).

Breathing
Think through the respiratory pathway:
● **Central drive**: see opiates above; major intracerebral events,
  subclinical status epilepticus.
● **Nerve transmission**: high spinal cord lesion usually due to trauma
  (consider this in the elderly rheumatoid patient who falls on the
  ward—immobilize the neck). Guillain–Barré syndrome.
● **Neuromuscular**: myasthenia, Eaton–Lambert, occasionally in the
  immediately post-operative patient with insufficient reversal.
● **Muscular**: some will be obvious, such as Duchenne's muscular
  dystrophy, but beware patients on large doses of dantrolene for MS
  and post-ICU patients.
● **Pulmonary**: most common:
  • Infection: if appropriate these patients are likely to need respiratory
    support.
  • Bronchospasm: 📖 section on Asthma, Chapter 20.
  • Pneumothorax: 📖 algorithm, Chapter 26.

Circulation
● **Non-cardiogenic**
  • Hypovolaemia.
  • Sepsis and vasodilatation.
  • Anaphylaxis.
  • Vasodilatory drugs.
● **Cardiogenic**
  • Intrinsic: ischaemia, valves, arrhythmia, failure.
  • Extrinsic: pulmonary embolus, tamponade.

Immediate actions
Airway
● Airway not compromised: continue below.
● Airway compromised: use simple manoeuvres, insert an oropharyngeal
  or nasopharyngeal airway.

- Remove foreign bodies if possible and visible, but remember good-fitting dentures may assist with maintaining an airway.
- Ensure suction is available, and switched on.
- Nominate an appropriate person to look after the airway; call for anaesthetic help if appropriate (see below).

Breathing

- Apply high-flow oxygen (☞ see opposite for discussion of chronic CO_2 retention and the peri-arrest patient).
- If signs of tension pneumothorax perform needle decompression, second intercostal space, mid-clavicular line; use an IV cannula at least 18G (📖 Chapter 26).
- If evidence of bronchospasm apply continuous beta-2 agonist nebulizers driven with oxygen.
- If conscious level is preserved but hypoxic or with pulmonary oedema consider early use of CPAP (📖 Chapter 47).
- Consider whether NIV is appropriate (COPD exacerbation, hypercapnia, pH < 7.35; 📖 Chapter 47).

⚠ Do not attempt to intubate a patient yourself who is not in cardio-respiratory arrest.
Call an anaesthetist (or ICU) if:
- Severe respiratory failure.
  - RR <10 or >30.
  - PaO_2 <10 on high-flow oxygen.
  - Rising $PaCO_2$ and acidosis.
- Decreased conscious level (AVPU P or U).
- Airway compromise, anatomical or oedema.
- Cardioversion needed and patient conscious (⚠ if your patient is severely compromised, e.g. hypotensive in VT with impaired conscious level and needs cardioversion, do not delay. Give 2–5 mg midazolam IV, increased if necessary in steps of 1 mg to a maximum of 7.5 mg, and cardiovert).

Circulation

- Get good IV access. A cannula in the external jugular vein is sometimes the most rapidly available route if peripheral veins cannot be accessed and gives short circulation times for resuscitation drugs.
- If symptomatic bradycardia give IV atropine 300–600 mcg (repeat as necessary to 3 mg and consider external pacing).
- Provided patient is not in heart failure and does not have intrinsic cardiogenic shock then give fluid challenge (250 ml colloid or 500 ml crystalloid) and repeat if beneficial and required.
- If the patient remains hypotensive then obtain central access and fill to a CVP of 8–12 cm. Vasoactive drugs may then be required.

✦ Hypercapnia and the peri-arrest patient

The majority of hypercapnic peri-arrest patients require high-flow oxygen; therefore if no medical information is available this treatment should be started. If the patient is known to have COPD with chronic hypoxia and chronic hypercapnia, titrate the O_2 concentration to the level required to achieve an SaO_2 of 85–90% using venturi adaptors. If the patient remains hypoxic, hypercapnic, and acidotic then they will need respiratory support (either NIV or intubation and ventilation).

Further circulatory management

▶▶ If your patient is extremely hypotensive (systolic <70 mmHg) while you are setting up your central access kit you may need to give very small boluses of peripheral vasopressors. Adrenaline is always available as 1:10 000 minijets (1 mg in 10 ml) on the arrest trolley and 0.5–1.0 ml (50–100 mcg) boluses can be given every 3–5 minutes to maintain a blood pressure. This can also be used in refractory bradycardia whilst setting up external pacing or obtaining equipment.

Vasoactive drugs are used to maintain a sensible perfusion pressure and hopefully cardiac output. Expertise is needed in using these and at this stage you should have the intensive care team to help. The following is provided as a reminder.

⚠ Must be via central line unless stated otherwise. Patients should have ECG monitoring continuously and invasive arterial pressure monitoring established as soon as possible: set non-invasive BP cuff to record every 3–5 minutes in the interim. Starting doses are assuming a 70 kg adult.

Vasoconstrictors

Noradrenaline

- Pure vasoconstriction (at usual doses) so will increase BP with little effect on cardiac output.
- Usually given as 40 mcg/ml 0.9% saline; start at 10–20 ml/hour and titrate upwards.

Metaraminol

- Pure vasoconstrictor. Slower onset and offset than noradrenaline so can be given in small boluses peripherally.
- Usually dilute 10 mg (1 ml ampoule) in 20 ml 0.9% saline and given in 1–2 ml aliquots.
- Often used to maintain BP at time of induction and intubation in sick patients.

Inoconstrictors: increase BP and cardiac output

Adrenaline

- As an infusion 5 ml of 1:10 000 at a rate of 1 ml (100 mcg)/minute.
- In extremis (see above) 10 ml from 1:10 000 minijet (1 mg).

Ephedrine

❶ *Do not confuse with adrenaline (see above).*
- Slower onset and longer lasting than adrenaline and much less potent.
- Usually dilute 30 mg (1 ml ampoule) in 10 ml 0.9% saline and give as bolus of 3 mg (1 ml).
- Often used at induction/intubation to maintain BP.

Dopamine

- Effects vary with dose. Can be given peripherally if diluted in 500 ml.
- Dilute to maximum of 3.2 mg/ml in 0.7% saline and infuse at 2–5 mcg/kg/minute.
- Low-dose dopamine for 'renal protection' is ineffective.
- It is still used as an inoconstrictor, although many units prefer to use other agents.

Inodilators

Dobutamine

- Will increase cardiac output and vasodilate, thereby offloading the myocardium and increasing peripheral perfusion. In some circumstances (underfilled, misdiagnosed sepsis) this will result in a dramatic fall in BP. Will increase both heart rate and contractility.
- Dilute to 0.5–1 mg/ml in 0.9% saline and infuse at 2.5–10 mcg/kg/minute.
- Often used (in conjunction with a constrictor such as noradrenaline) to improve tissue perfusion, as inferred from central venous oxygen saturations (see below).

Vasodilators

GTN

- Used to treat refractory angina or LVF.
- Boluses given sublingually (usually 500 µg).
- As an infusion 100–400 mcg/ml in 0.9% saline and infuse at 10–200 mcg/minute if required. Tolerance develops over 24–48 hours of continuous infusion.

Ongoing management

Ideally by this stage the patient is becoming stable and you have worked out the cause of the deterioration and initiated appropriate treatment. You should have the results of capillary glucose, CXR, ABG, and 12-lead ECG, and formal bloods should be on their way. If the diagnosis remains elusive, try to obtain an emergency echocardiogram. This will tell you:
- LV size and function.
- Rule out tamponade and acute valvular dysfunction.
- Regional wall motion abnormalities which may suggest ischaemia.
- May inform you about pulmonary artery pressures and RV function.
- Will occasionally show direct evidence of pulmonary embolism such as thrombus in transit.

This patient is clearly sick and likely to benefit from level 2 or 3 care, which in most hospitals will involve liaison with the intensive care team.

Other investigations

Will be suggested by your findings; for example, a history suggestive of PE will prompt an echo or CT pulmonary angiogram, focal neurology and decreased conscious level will suggest CT head, an infarct on ECG will suggest thrombolysis and transfer to CCU.

⚠ Do not attempt to transfer the patient to the CT scanner or high dependency unit without achieving stability, ensuring adequate monitoring and having appropriately trained staff. Again this will often involve liaison with the ICU team.

Targets

Normality is often difficult to achieve so what is reasonable in the short term when stabilizing the peri-arrest patient? The following are a guide.

- RR <25.
- SaO_2 >90% (lower if COPD).
- HR 60–100 (accept outside this if other parameters acceptable).
- Mean arterial pressure >65 mmHg (higher if chronic hypertension).
- CVP 8–12 (or >3 cm above baseline pre-resuscitation and sustained).
- Capillary refill time <2 seconds.
- Urine output >0.5 ml/kg/hour.
- Normal conscious level.
- Arterial pH >7.25.
- Lactate <2.0 mmol/L (higher suggests poor perfusion).
- Central venous oxygen saturation ($ScvO_2$) >70%.

Driving targets beyond this is unlikely to give incremental benefit.

Dyspnoea

① Dyspnoea

The American Thoracic Society defines dyspnoea as 'a term used to characterize a subjective experience of breathing discomfort that is comprised of qualitatively distinct sensations that vary in intensity. The experience derives from interactions among multiple physiological, psychological, social and environmental factors and may include secondary physiological and behavioural responses.'

Dyspnoea is a common symptom and the presenting complaint of the majority of patients with respiratory disease. Acute dyspnoea usually comes on over the course of minutes to hours. Associated symptoms and signs may help with clues to the aetiology. Chronic dyspnoea occurs in the majority of respiratory conditions, the commonest being COPD and interstitial lung disease, as well as a number of cardiac conditions.

In many respiratory conditions causing chronic dyspnoea, patients will present with acute on chronic dyspnoea due to an exacerbation of their underlying condition, superimposed infection, a complication of their existing disease, such as pneumothorax or PE, or unrelated pathology.

Many causes of dyspnoea present with a normal CXR and this should not rule out a respiratory cause.

Causes of acute dyspnoea

Respiratory

- Acute asthma.
- Exacerbation of COPD (often occurs on a background of chronic dyspnoea).
- Pneumonia.
- Pneumothorax.
- Pulmonary embolus.
- Acute hypersensitivity pneumonitis.
- Hyperventilation: need to exclude underlying cause.

Cardiovascular

- Pulmonary oedema.
- Arrhythmia.
- Cardiac tamponade.

Other

- Anaphylaxis.
- Metabolic acidosis.
- Salicylate overdose.

Causes of subacute dyspnoea

Recent onset dyspnoea (days, weeks) may precede admission to hospital. This makes new sub-acute conditions more likely and includes those listed above plus the following.

Respiratory

- Pleural effusion.
- Lung malignancy.

- Exacerbation of bronchiectasis/cystic fibrosis.
- Cryptogenic organizing pneumonia.
- Acute interstitial pneumonia.
- Pulmonary vasculitis.
- Lymphangitis carcinomatosis.

Cardiovascular
- Congestive cardiac failure.
- Myocarditis.
- SVCO.

Other
- Anaemia.
- Thyrotoxicosis.

Causes of chronic dyspnoea

Chronic dyspnoea may be the presenting feature to the emergency department, but more usually presents as an acute worsening on a background of chronicity. Chronic episodic shortness of breath is more likely to occur in asthma, hypersensitivity pneumonitis, pulmonary embolism or cardiovascular causes.

Respiratory
- COPD.
- Chronic asthma.
- Interstitial lung disease including IPF and sarcoid.
- Pleural effusion.
- Bronchiectasis/cystic fibrosis.
- Lung malignancy.
- Obliterative bronchiolitis.

Cardiovascular
- Congestive cardiac failure.
- Cardiomyopathy.
- Valvular disease.
- Pulmonary hypertension (primary and secondary).
- Shunt (intracardiac or intrapulmonary).

Other
- Neuromuscular disease.
- Anaemia.
- Thyrotoxicosis.

Assessing the patient

History, examination and investigation will narrow down the differential diagnosis.

History
- Ask the patient to describe the character of their shortness of breath. Often they are unable to do this, but certain associated factors such as a description of chest tightness may point to the underlying problem.
- Duration and speed of onset: pneumothorax and pulmonary embolus are the usual causes of instantaneous shortness of breath.

- Usual exercise tolerance. It is helpful to ask the patient about their normal functional status. Are they breathless at the top of one flight of stairs? Also, how does this compare with 1 week or 6 months ago? This will give information on whether there is likely to be an underlying lung disease and the speed of onset of their condition.
- Severity of dyspnoea.
- Explore associated features such as wheeze, peripheral oedema, fever, cough, haemoptysis, or chest pain. If pleuritic pain consider pneumothorax, PE, or pneumonia, compared with retrosternal chest pain which may make pulmonary oedema a more likely diagnosis. In acute dyspnoea associated with wheeze, the presence of urticaria may help differentiate between anaphylaxis and asthma.
- Exacerbating features or triggers, such as cold or exercise with asthma, orthopnoea, and nocturnal breathlessness with left ventricular failure. Breathlessness on swimming or in the bath is commonly associated with diaphragmatic paralysis.
- Past medical and family history of chest disease.
- Review smoking history, drug use, occupational history and other exposure history.
- Review medications. Has the patient stopped or run out of usual medication or been started on new medication such as beta-blockers or NSAIDs that may aggravate underlying asthma?
- In older patients with more complex medical histories the onset of dyspnoea may well be multifactorial and not simply due to a single disease process.

Examination

Note respiratory rate, pattern of breathing, use of accessory muscles, and paradoxical abdominal movement (in diaphragmatic paralysis).

Examine for clubbing, cyanosis, asterixis, lymphadenopathy, and evidence of SVCO (facial swelling, distended neck veins, collaterals over chest wall). Examine legs for swelling and or tenderness.

Full examination of cardiovascular and respiratory systems.

Investigations

- SaO_2
- Peak flow
- FBC
- CXR
- ABG
- ECG

Consider further investigations as appropriate.

- Further blood tests (such as TFTs, cardiac enzymes, vasculitic screen, etc.).
- Exercise oximetry.
- CT chest (HRCT/CTPA).
- Plasma BNP in the investigation of cardiac failure.
- Pulmonary function tests (± reversibility testing).
- ECHO.
- Coronary angiography.

Wheeze and dyspnoea

Introduction

A wheeze is a continuous musical sound that may be mono- or polyphonic in nature, depending on its cause, and may originate from an airway of any size. It is produced by oscillation of opposing walls of a narrowed airway and is typically described in expiration. Stridor is the term used for an inspiratory noise, most commonly over the central airways, and is discussed in Chapter 42.

The most common cause of acute wheeze and dyspnoea is asthma; however, there is a large differential diagnosis to be considered. A useful approach is to divide the causes of wheeze and dyspnoea as to whether they occur in the upper or lower airway.

:✪: Causes of wheeze and dyspnoea

Upper airway
- Anaphylaxis: abrupt onset of wheeze and dyspnoea with urticaria and/or angioedema. Often history of insect bite or consumption of food or drug. May have had prior episodes or a positive family history.
- Epiglottitis: more commonly causes stridor and drooling. Sore throat out of proportion to visible pharyngitis. ❶ Urgent referral to ENT.
- Vocal cord dysfunction: Severe symptoms in absence of increased A–a gradient. Lack of response to bronchodilators. Variable flow–volume loops. Paradoxical movement of vocal cords on laryngoscopy during wheezing. ❶ Often coexists with asthma.
- Neoplasm: more commonly associated with stridor.

Lower airway
- Asthma: episodic, triggering factors, family history. Responds to bronchodilators.
- COPD: SOB on exertion, may have chronic productive cough, smoking history, irreversible airflow obstruction on spirometry.
- Pulmonary oedema: History of cardiac disease, chest pain, cardiac risk factors. Orthopnoea and PND.
- Bronchiectasis: Chronic productive purulent cough, episodes of fever or recurrent infections. Coarse crackles present in addition to wheeze. Crackles often inspiratory and expiratory and do not change on coughing.
- Allergic bronchopulmonary aspergillosis: deterioration in asthmatic patient. Associated eosinophilia and raised IgE. Segmental or lobar collapse may be seen on CXR.
- Cystic fibrosis: likely to be a known diagnosis but can present later in adulthood. Clubbed, bronchiectasis, progressive obstructive lung disease. May have associated pancreatic insufficiency with low BMI, stunted growth. Family history.
- Neoplasms: particularly with unilateral wheeze. May be associated with haemoptysis, smoking history, and CXR changes (particularly lobar collapse if airway obstruction is present).

- Lymphangitis carcinomatosis – Either in patient with known malignancy or occasionally as first presentation of malignancy. Abnormal CXR.
- Carcinoid syndrome – episodic flushing and diarrhoea associated with wheeze. Check 24 hour urinary 5-HIAA.
- Parasitic infection – history of travel to endemic area. Associated fever, weight loss and peripheral blood eosinophilia. Stool and blood serology for diagnosis.

History and examination

- Episodic wheezing, often associated with dyspnoea and cough, should direct the diagnosis towards asthma. Symptoms should respond to inhaled or nebulized bronchodilators.
- Review exacerbating or triggering factors.
- Acute onset of nocturnal dyspnoea associated with wheeze may represent pulmonary oedema. Associated chest pain or cardiac risk factors may provide additional clues, as may evidence of peripheral oedema.
- Unilateral monophonic wheeze should raise suspicion of airway obstruction, for example by foreign body or malignancy.
- Past medical (including past chest) history and family history (especially for asthma).
- Smoking and drug history, occupational or recreational exposure history, and medications.
- Visual examination of upper airway should be performed along with palpation of neck for extra-thoracic obstruction and examination of the cardiac and respiratory systems.

Investigations

Initial

- SaO_2.
- HR, RR, temperature, blood pressure.
- Peak flow.
- FBC.
- CXR.
- ECG.
- ABG if SaO_2 <92%, or in COPD and concerns re hypercapnia.
- Simple spirometry if available.

Later investigation as applicable

- Pulmonary function tests.
- Plasma BNP or ECHO.
- CT chest.

Initial management
- Oxygen.
- Nebulized bronchodilator.
- Consider oral steroid.
- Consider antihistamine and adrenaline (IM) if evidence of anaphylaxis.
- Treatment of underlying cause.

Chapter 4

Dyspnoea in specific situations

☼ Dyspnoea in the post-operative patient

May be due to:

- Exacerbation of an existing condition, such as asthma or COPD.
- A new condition, e.g. cardiac arrhythmia.
- The operation itself, particularly with upper GI or thoracic surgery.
- Anaesthesia and immobility.

The initial assessment of the patient should be aimed at resuscitation and treatment, particularly the need for ITU care and ventilation.

Causes

Immediate

▶ *Exclude upper airway obstruction first (*📖 *Chapter 42).*

- Pulmonary oedema: secondary to fluid overload in patients with limited myocardial reserve, ischaemic myocardial damage, arrhythmias.
- Aspiration pneumonitis: more common in intestinal obstruction and pregnancy.
- Pulmonary embolism (consider fat and air embolism).
- Anaesthetic effect or opiate excess, causing respiratory depression.

Later

- Atelectasis: particularly following abdominal and thoracic surgery. Usually within 48 hours and more common in the elderly, COPD, smokers, and obese patients. May get lobar collapse.
- Pulmonary oedema due to fluid overload or ischaemic heart disease/arrhythmia (usually AF).
- Post-operative pneumonia: more common if aspiration/atelectasis/copious secretions. Often gram-negative bacteria.
- Pulmonary embolism, particularly pelvic procedures/known malignancy/previous VTE.
- Exacerbation of underlying pulmonary condition such as COPD.
- Anaemia.
- ARDS.
- Metabolic acidosis, usually due to renal failure or sepsis.

Investigations

- Routine bloods including FBC, U&E, LFT, and CRP (though CRP often elevated secondary to operation). D-dimer will not help as it will be raised post-operatively with or without thromboembolism.
- ECG.
- CXR.
- ABG.

Management

Entirely dependent on cause.

Basal atelectasis

Appropriate analgesia to aid coughing, chest physiotherapy ± saline nebulizers to help expectoration.

Pneumonia

Treat with high-flow oxygen, fluid resuscitation if required, broad-spectrum antibiotics and chest physiotherapy. Use antibiotics for hospital-acquired infection to cover Gram-negative organisms (📖 Chapter 27, pneumonia) and consider covering for aspiration.

Pulmonary embolism

If patient is hypoxic with raised A–a gradient (📖 Chapter 53) and no evident cause on CXR, then proceed to CTPA. Treat with full-dose LMWH if no contraindications (will depend on surgical procedure).

Pulmonary oedema

Treat with oxygen, diuretics ± nitrite infusion. Central line and inotropes may be required. Investigate cause: fluid overload, myocardial damage, arrhythmia. Perform ECG, consider cardiac enzymes, tight fluid balance, echocardiogram.

Respiratory failure

If there is evidence of type 2 respiratory failure with no overt cause consider anaesthetic agents or opiate excess (trial naloxone 400 mcg IV). Calculating the A–a gradient may be helpful in distinguishing neuromuscular causes ('pump failure') from pulmonary disease impairing gas exchange (📖 Chapter 8).

Consider precipitation of myaesthenic crisis following anaesthetic agents: intubate and ventilate, send acetylcholine receptor antibodies and treat with IV immunoglobulin.

Look for evidence of pre-existing pulmonary pathology such as COPD and treat appropriately.

Anaemia

Exclude any ongoing bleeding. Cross match and transfuse.

:⊙: Dyspnoea in pregnancy

Dyspnoea during pregnancy is common, with approximately 60% of women complaining of exertional dyspnoea whilst 20% report dyspnoea at rest. Both physiological and hormonal factors contribute to dyspnoea (see below). Distinguishing this 'physiological dyspnoea' from specific coexisting conditions or disorders complicating pregnancy is essential.

Normal physiological changes in pregnancy
Anatomical changes

In normal pregnancy there is a reduction in the functional residual capacity and residual volume due to an upward movement of the diaphragm by approximately 4 cm. There is an associated increase in vital capacity; however, total lung capacity and FEV_1 remain unchanged.

Ventilation

Minute ventilation increases because of stimulation by elevated progesterone levels and the PaO_2 increases. Pregnant women usually mildly hyperventilate to maintain a low $PaCO_2$ in order to maintain a gradient for CO_2 diffusion from fetal blood. In addition, cardiac output increases by up to 40% and plasma volume by up to 50%.

Haemodynamic changes

Progressive increase in cardiac output from the first trimester; up to 40% above baseline by the third trimester.

Thrombotic state

Increased coagulation factors and venous stasis of the pelvic veins leads to a fivefold increased risk of thromboembolism, which is a major cause of maternal death.

Causes of SOB in pregnancy
Pulmonary
- Exacerbation or worsening of pre-existing condition, e.g. asthma, bronchiectasis, pulmonary hypertension.
- Pulmonary embolism.
- Aspiration pneumonitis.
- Pneumothorax.
- Pleural effusion: can be seen in the post-partum period and rarely in ovarian hyperstimulation syndrome (following IVF).

Cardiac
- Valvular heart disease (may previously have been undiagnosed and precipitated by increased cardiac output).
- ▶ Undiagnosed mitral stenosis can cause pulmonary oedema in labour.
- Cardiomyopathy.

Other
- ARDS: associated with obstetric complications e.g. amniotic fluid embolus, placental abruption, eclampsia, or non-obstetric conditions which are more common in pregnancy, e.g. gastric aspiration, sepsis (pelvic and non-pelvic), and massive haemorrhage.
- Anaemia.

Pregnancy-specific disorders

- Amniotic fluid embolization (rare, 1 in 25 000). High mortality.
- Tocolytic pulmonary oedema (caused by beta-adrenergic agonists used to inhibit pre-term labour).
- Pre-eclampsia and pulmonary oedema.
- Peri-partum cardiomyopathy (usually develops in the last month of pregnancy).

Asthma in pregnancy

Approximately a third become worse, a third become better and a third stay the same. Asthma deterioration is often between weeks 24 and 36.

Asthma is associated with an increased risk of pre-eclampsia. However, studies have shown that increased asthma symptoms and poor control both before and during pregnancy lead to this increased risk, as opposed to asthma alone.

Asthma is also associated with an increased risk of intra-uterine growth retardation (IUGR). Again, studies have shown that those with well-controlled asthma (relatively asymptomatic, GINA 1) have no or minimal IUGR, with increasing IUGR as control or symptoms worsen.

There are often compliance issues with asthma medications during pregnancy as women are concerned about the possible effects on the fetus. Asthma medications, including oral steroids, are generally regarded as safe in pregnancy and should be continued.

▶ Poor control is more harmful to the mother and fetus than asthma medication.

Acute asthma in pregnancy

- Treat as for the non-pregnant asthmatic (📖 Chapter 20).
- GORD often a trigger factor for asthma and this increases in pregnancy.
- Maintain SaO_2 >95% to prevent fetal hypoxia.
- Monitor fetus in severe asthma and liaise with obstetricians.

Drugs

All common asthma medications can be continued in pregnancy (beta-2 agonists, inhaled corticosteroids, long-acting beta-agonists, theophylline) except for the newer leukotriene receptor antagonists where there is little data on their use in pregnancy. However, if the mother has good control on a leukotriene receptor antagonist then they should be continued in pregnancy, as worsening control will do more harm.

Labour

Because of increased release of endogenous steroid it is very rare to have an acute exacerbation of asthma during labour.

Prostaglandin E_2 may be safely used in induction of labour, whilst prostaglandin F_2 alpha, used in post-partum haemorrhage, may cause bronchospasm.

Use IV hydrocortisone 100 mg 6–8 hourly during labour in those who have been taking >7.5 mg oral prednisolone for >2 weeks before delivery.

Pulmonary embolism in pregnancy

Despite increased awareness, this remains the most common cause of maternal death and mortality still occurs because of lack of recognition and timely diagnosis.

There is an increased risk of thromboembolism in pregnancy because of

- increased coagulability.
- increased venous stasis: >30% reduction in flow by 15/40 weeks, >60% by 36/40 weeks.

Ileofemoral deep vein thrombosis (DVT) occurs more commonly than popliteofemoral DVT in pregnancy and is far more frequent than in the non-pregnant population. Pregnancy is also a risk factor for recurrent DVT, with a threefold increase in relative risk.

Increased risk of pulmonary embolism

- Age >35 years.
- Caesarian section.
- Increased BMI.
- Positive family history or known thrombophilia.
- Previous thrombosis.
- Pre-eclampsia.

Investigation of PE in pregnancy

If there is clinical suspicion of PE, D-dimer will not add to the investigation as it is usually raised in normal pregnancy ($\Box$ p. 184 *PE algorithm*). The negative predictive value is also less reliable in pregnancy.

Ideally, the first investigation of choice should be bilateral leg USS. This involves no radiation exposure to the mother or fetus and if positive precludes the need for further investigation.

The choice of further investigation is between CTPA and ventilation–perfusion scan. Radiation doses are as follows.

- Perfusion scan exposes the fetus to <0.12mGy.
- Ventilation scan <0.35mGy.
- CXR <0.1mGy.

A CTPA gives a radiation dose to the fetus that is less than that of a V/Q scan, but an increased exposure to the mother which increases the lifetime risk of breast cancer in the mother by 14%. On the basis of this, the investigation of choice in those with a normal CXR is a perfusion scan.

Treatment of PE

- Requires a minimum of 3 months anticoagulation.
- Avoid warfarin: teratogenic to the fetus and increased risk of maternal haemorrhage.
- Low molecular weight heparin (LMWH) is the anticoagulant of choice, with a switch to unfractionated heparin for the delivery. Levels of LMWH can be monitored with anti-Xa levels (0.4–1.2 U/ml therapeutic anticoagulation).
- Anticoagulation should be continued throughout the pregnancy and for at least 6 weeks post-partum or until 3 months treatment has been completed.
- Pregnancy is not a contraindication to thrombolysis for massive PE.

Other pre-existing pulmonary conditions in pregnancy

Pulmonary hypertension

Pregnancy occurring in those with pulmonary hypertension has an associated high mortality, up to 30–50%. Increased cardiac output precipitates right heart failure. IUGR occurs in >30%. Echocardiography does not reliably measure pulmonary artery pressure in pregnancy.

Cystic fibrosis

In those with FEV_1 >60% predicted, there is no increased mortality associated with pregnancy. In those with more severe disease the outcome is poor, with increased perinatal mortality due to pre-term delivery or complications of CF.

Lymphangioleiomyomatosis

Often presents for the first time in pregnancy; otherwise worsens in pregnancy as the disease process (abnormal proliferation of smooth muscle cells) is driven by oestrogen. Common presentations include dyspnoea, cough, pneumothorax, and pleural effusion (particularly chylothorax).

① Dyspnoea and fever in the returning traveller

Both travel abroad by UK residents and the number of visitors and immigrants from abroad are increasing year by year, and therefore this is becoming an increasingly common presentation to A&E.

Approximately half of those presenting after recent travel will have a non-tropical cause for their fever and shortness of breath (e.g. community acquired pneumonia). In returning travellers from tropical areas, malaria is by far the most common cause of fever.

Cause of infection is dependent on the location and duration of travel. Differential diagnosis can be further narrowed down by considering exposure history, relevant incubation period, and findings.

History
- Country travelled to and stopovers.
- Duration of travel.
- Accommodation, i.e. hotel, camping.
- Food and water consumed, i.e. fresh, bottled, tinned.
- Any insect or animal bites.
- Domestic pets.
- Leisure activities, e.g. watersports.
- Occupation.
- Vaccinations and prophylaxis.
- Sexual activity, IV drug use, tattooing, transfusions.
- Contacts with unwell people.
- PMH.

Examination
Full systemic examination.
Look in particular for skin and genital lesions, conjunctival change, lymphadenopathy, liver and spleen.

Investigations
- FBC, U&E, LFTs, CRP.
- Thick and thin films for malaria.
- Serology.
- Urinalysis and MSU.
- Blood cultures.
- Stool culture if appropriate.
- CXR.
- Further imaging: USS/CT.
- Specific tests for a suspected diagnosis: antibody titres, immunological investigations.

Causes

More frequent

- Community-acquired pneumonia.
- Mycoplasma
  - Atypical pneumonia. Often presents with dry cough, headache, diarrhoea, anaemia (cold agglutinin), and abnormal LFT.
- *Legionella*
  - Outbreaks in hotels with contaminated cooling systems.
  - Incubation 2–10 days.
  - Prodromal viral-like illness; then dry cough, tachypnoea, diarrhoea and confusion.
  - Lymphopaenia and hyponatraemia seen.
  - Diagnosis: urinary *Legionella* antigen ± serology.
  - Treatment with macrolides ± rifampicin.
- Tuberculosis
  - Contact history, often productive cough with fevers, sweats and weight loss. Abnormal CXR. Be aware of extrapulmonary tuberculosis.
- Typhoid
  - Insidious onset with headache and fever, then cough, rash (rose-spots), and constipation. Later get diarrhoea, pneumonia, and other complications.
  - Diagnosis: blood cultures early, urine and stool cultures later.
  - Treatment with ciprofloxacin.
- Viral pneumonia.

Less common

- Q fever
  - Caused by *Coxiella burnetii*. Infection by inhalation (increased risk with farmyard exposure). Incubation 2–3 weeks.
  - Fever, myalgia, dry cough, GI symptoms, and chest pain. 30–50% develop pneumonia.
  - Diagnosis on serology. Treat with doxycycline.
- Diptheria
  - Epidemic in Russia and Eastern Europe.
  - Incubation 2–5 days.
  - Laryngeal diphtheria gives husky voice, cough, and later dyspnoea and stridor due to respiratory obstruction. Usually cervical lymph nodes (giving 'bull neck') and pharyngeal membrane (greyish yellow) present.
  - Diagnosis usually clinical (send cultures and serology). Treat with anti-toxin and macrolide or penicillin.
- Pertussis
  - 90% of cases occur in children <5 years of age but can affect any age.
  - Initially malaise, then characteristic paroxysms of coughing; 'whoop' characteristically in children.
  - Diagnosis by culture of nasopharyngeal secretions, treat with macrolides.

- Anthrax
  - Occurs worldwide.
  - Transmission through direct contact with infected animal.
  - Inhalation of spores results in dry cough and fever with chest discomfort for 2–3 days; then dramatic deterioration with dyspnoea and hypoxia.
  - CXR shows widened mediastinum (due to haemorrhagic mediastinits) or pleural effusion.
  - Diagnosed by culture (Gram-positive rod) or fourfold antibody rise. Treat with penicillin or macrolides, drain pleural fluid.
- Tularaemia
  - Worldwide, but frequently seen in USA.
  - Transmission via handling infected meat or tick bite.
  - Pneumonic form.
  - Diagnose on culture and treat with gentamicin.
- Meliodosis
  - Penetrates skin abrasions: usually seen in those who go barefoot, e.g. paddy-field farmers in Southeast Asia.
  - Acute septicaemia with lung, kidney, and liver involvement or chronic pneumonic form. CXR may resemble TB.
  - Diagnose on culture; treat with ceftazidime.
- Botulism
  - *Clostridium botulinum* proliferates in preserved canned foods.
  - Toxins cause neuromuscular blockade, with neurological symptoms dominating and respiratory insufficiency occurring.
  - Toxin detected in serum or faeces.
  - Anti-toxin and supportive treatment.
- Brucellosis
  - Worldwide zoonosis.
  - Infection through unpasteurised milk.
  - Usually undulating fever, malaise, and night sweats. Localized brucellosis in the lung (with systemic symptoms in a third) is uncommon.
  - Diagnose on culture or serology. Treat with doxycycline and rifampicin.

Chapter 5

Cough, sputum, and fever

⊕ Cough, sputum, and fever

The development of the combination of a cough, sputum production, and a fever usually implies pulmonary infection of some form. It may be a new infection in otherwise normal lungs, e.g. pneumonia, or the worsening of a chronic disease, e.g. bronchiectasis or COPD. The assessment of the patient follows the standard format.

History

A full history should be taken from the patient and/or relatives as soon as the situation is sufficiently stable to do so.

- Cough: acute/chronic.
- Sputum
  - Acute/chronic, able to expectorate, purulent, associated haemoptysis.
  - If chronic, what is normal volume, colour, consistency?
  - Streaky haemoptysis common in CF and bronchiectasis.
- Fever, rigors, night sweats.
- Other symptoms
  - Dyspnoea, chest pain, wheeze, malaise, weight loss.
- Previous medical history
  - Prior cardiorespiratory disease.
  - Immunosuppression: disease related or iatrogenic.
- Prior medications
  - May indicate chronic respiratory disease.
  - Prior antibiotic use: determine which antibiotics have previously improved symptoms. If previous lack of response to oral antibiotics, consider *Pseudomonas* infection.
- Allergies
  - Penicillin allergy and if present its nature. Many patients with 'penicillin allergy' will be able to tolerate cephalosporins.
- Travel
  - Risks for TB, *Legionella*.
- Smoking.
- Alcohol.
- Pets: in particular whether the patient keeps birds.
- Family history.

Examination

- General
  - How unwell is the patient? The initial end of the bed assessment of the acute patient should guide subsequent actions.
- Respiratory
  - Airway.
  - Respiratory rate and effort.
  - Cyanosis: peripheral or central.
  - Evidence of chronic lung disease, e.g. hyperinflation, clubbing.
  - Expansion, percussion, auscultation. Presence of secretions, consolidation or pleural fluid.

- Circulation
  - Evidence of sepsis (hypotension, tachycardia).
  - Urine output and fluid balance.
- Neurological assessment
  - Look for reasons for aspiration pneumonia: depressed conscious level, dysphasia, dysphagia, stroke, neuromuscular disease. If suspected, the patient should remain nil by mouth until formal assessment is possible.

Investigations

- Temperature, heart rate, blood pressure, respiratory rate.
- Oxygen saturation.
- Blood glucose.
- ECG.
- Bloods including FBC (note WCC including eosinophils), U&Es, LFTs.
- CRP.
- Clotting screen: coagulopathy of sepsis or DIC.
- Blood cultures prior to antibiotics.
- CXR.
- Arterial blood gas.
- Sputum cultures in:
  - Chronic respiratory disease where bacterial pathogen is uncertain or when antibiotic resistance is suspected, e.g. CF and bronchiectasis.
  - Suspected TB (three samples for AFB).
- Urinary antigen tests to identify bacterial antigens in urine. They can provide rapid results, helping guide diagnosis and therapy even if performed after the initiation of antibiotic therapy. There are two commonly performed tests.

Legionella urinary antigen
  - Most *Legionella* pneumonia (80%) is caused by *Legionella pneumophila* serogroup 1. *Legionella* pneumonia is more likely to cause severe community-acquired pneumonia (CAP).
  - Some laboratories only test for serogroup 1 and so it is important to know what test your local laboratory uses as a negative result does not exclude *Legionella*.

Pneumococcal urinary antigen
  - Streptococcus pneumoniae antigen can be detected in the urine.
  - Individual hospitals will have their own policies for use of these tests. The BTS recommends both *Legionella* urinary antigen and pneumococcal urinary antigen are performed in severe community-acquired pneumonia.
- Serology for atypical pathogens
  - Change in IgG and IgM titre in paired blood samples (taken when ill and convalescing) can prove infection.
  - *Legionella pneumophila*, *Mycoplasma*, and *Chlamydia pneumoniae* are the usual pathogens tested for.

- No use in initial management of the acutely unwell patient in whom urinary antigen testing is preferred.
- Criteria for performing these tests depend on the requirement for microbiological surveillance and are usually agreed locally between clinicians, laboratory staff, and public health officers.
- Diagnostic pleural aspiration if a pleural effusion is present.
  - pH, protein, LDH, glucose, MC & S, AFBs.
- Bronchoscopy
  - Rarely needed in the acute setting for diagnosis. It should be considered in the immunocompromised (if they are stable enough for it to be done safely), as the potential pathogens are more varied, or if aspiration of a foreign body is suspected.

Differential diagnosis
- Pneumonia
  - Bacterial.
  - Viral.
  - Fungal.
- Acute bronchitis.
- Acute exacerbation of COPD.
- Acute exacerbation of known bronchiectasis/CF.
- Mycobacterial disease
  - TB.
  - Non-tuberculous *Mycobacterium*.
- Cryptogenic organizing pneumonia (COP).
- Eosinophilic pneumonia.
- Hypersensitivity pneumonitis (extrinsic allergic alveolitis).
- Allergic bronchopulmonary aspergillosis (ABPA).

Management

Severity assessment
Initial care should be guided by:
- Heart rate, blood pressure, respiratory rate, temperature.
- Oxygen saturation.
- ABG: oxygenation, ventilation, and tissue perfusion via serum lactate.
- Neurological status: GCS, confusion.
- Circulation and intravascular volume status.
In community-acquired pneumonia there are several proposed severity assessment scores. The CURB-65 score is described in 📖 Chapter 27.

The basis of the treatment of pneumonia and other forms of pulmonary infection follows the basic scheme for all acute scenarios. It consists of:
- The immediate recognition of any life-threatening conditions and their prompt correction (📖 Chapter 1).
- ABC.

- Oxygen: ensure adequate arterial levels to help maintain O_2 delivery to the tissues.
  - Most patients with pneumonia have type 1 respiratory failure, but may present with acute type 2 respiratory failure (📖 Chapter 8). They are best helped by providing a FiO_2 that maintains an adequate arterial oxygen level. Acute hypercapnia and respiratory acidosis with a normal base excess implies acute ventilatory failure and should prompt consideration of ICU care.
  - Limiting the FiO_2 may be appropriate for some COPD patients for whom oxygen genuinely does depress minute ventilation. An acute respiratory acidosis should be closely monitored alongside maximal therapy and assisted ventilation considered.
  - Consider NIV (📖 Chapter 47).
- Treat underlying condition:
  - Pneumonia—follow BTS guidelines (📖 Chapter 27).
  - Exacerbation of COPD (📖 Chapter 21).
  - Exacerbation of bronchiectasis (📖 Chapter 31).
  - Exacerbation of cystic fibrosis (📖 Chapter 32).
  - Immunocompromised (📖 Chapter 13).
- Regular observations
  - Assess response to therapy with monitoring of temperature, blood pressure, heart rate, oxygen saturation, and urine output. Can be used as 'early warning scores'.
- Nutrition.
- Physiotherapy.
  - Effective airway clearance crucial in bronchiectasis (📖 Chapter 50).

Further reading

1. 📖 Chapter 20, Bacterial respiratory infection, OHRM.
2. Rivers E et al. (2001). Early goal directed therapy in the treatment of severe sepsis and septic shock. N Engl J Med **345**, 1368–77.
3. Dellinger RP et al. (2004). Surviving sepsis campaign guidelines for management of severe sepsis and septic shock. Crit Care Med **32**, 858–73.

Haemoptysis

⚙ Haemoptysis

Haemoptysis refers to the expectoration of blood or blood-stained sputum.

Causes
Respiratory
- Bronchial carcinoma
- Pneumonia
- TB
- Cystic fibrosis
- Bronchiectasis
- Aspergilloma

Vascular/CVS
- Pulmonary embolism
- Mitral stenosis
- Arteriovenous malformation
- Hereditary haemorrhagic telangiectasia
- Pulmonary oedema

Iatrogenic
- Post bronchoscopy
- Post instrumentation

Vasculitis
- Wegener's granulomatosis
- Goodpasture's syndrome

Other
- Invading oesophageal carcinoma
- Clotting disorders
- Anti-coagulant therapy
- Endometriosis
- Upper airway origin of blood

History
- Is it blood alone or blood mixed with sputum? Colour of sputum?
  - Pulmonary oedema classically present pink frothy sputum. Bronchiectasis and pneumonia usually present with blood mixed with sputum.
- Chronicity of symptoms/previous episodes.
  - Points towards chronic condition, e.g. bronchiectasis, cystic fibrosis.
- Amount of blood.
  - Aspergilloma, vasculitis, AVM, cystic fibrosis, invading cancer most likely to cause massive haemoptysis.
- Time of occurrence of haemoptysis.
  - Occurring particularly after lying down is suggestive of an upper airway origin. Occurring with menstruation is suggestive of endometriosis.

- Associated symptoms.
  - Acute SOB and chest pain makes pneumonia or pulmonary embolism more likely, although SOB alone points toward pulmonary oedema. Progressive SOB more suggestive of mitral stenosis.
  - Fevers associated with weight loss occur in TB, although weight loss without fever may indicate lung cancer.
- Other sites of bleeding.
  - Haematuria occurring in vasculitis.
  - Epistaxis suggestive of Wegener's granulomatosis or hereditary haemorrhagic telangiectasia.
- Thorough PMH and drug history.

Examination

Inspection

- Cachexia: TB, cancer.
- Clubbing: bronchiectasis, lung cancer.
- Nasal passages (crusting) and saddling of nose in Wegener's granulomatosis.
- Malar flush.
- Telangiectasia.
- Raised JVP, peripheral oedema.
- Swollen face and distended veins with SVCO associated with cancer.
- Scars: previous surgery for lung cancer or bronchiectasis, chest drain scars.

Palpation

- Pulse rate and rhythm: tachycardia associated with infection and PE; AF associated with mitral stenosis and anticoagulation.
- Lymphadenopathy: infection (particularly TB) and cancer.
- Calf swelling and tenderness.

Auscultation

- Crackles: generally fine inspiratory with pulmonary oedema; coarse with infection or bronchiectasis.
- Bronchial breathing: infection.
- Decreased breath sounds/dull percussion note: effusion may point to cancer, TB or pneumonia, cardiac failure (more commonly bilateral), or pulmonary embolism.
- Diastolic murmur of mitral stenosis.

Investigations

- FBC.
- U&E.
- Clotting screen.
- Urine dip (proteinuria and haematuria in vasculitis).
- ECG.
- CXR.

- Arterial blood gas if SaO_2 <95%.
- Sputum for MC&S (and AFBs if suspected).
- ESR/CRP.

Specific investigations
- ANCA and antiglomerular basement membrane antibody if vasculitis suspected.
- *Aspergillus* precipitins (strongly positive in aspergilloma) and specific IgE to *Aspergillus*.
- Mantoux test if TB suspected.
- Bronchoscopy.
- CT chest: type dependent on suspicion (discuss with radiologist) to investigate PE, cancer, AVM, bronchiectasis.
- Bronchial angiography.
- Echocardiography if investigating mitral stenosis or pulmonary hypertension as the suspected cause of haemoptysis.

Management
- ABC.
- IV access (large bore if massive haemoptysis).
- Bloods including FBC, renal function, liver function, and clotting. Urgent cross-match if massive haemoptysis.
- Reverse anticoagulants.
- CXR.
- CT chest (unlikely to be possible in massive haemoptysis).

Small-volume haemoptysis
- As above.
- Start antibiotics if evidence of infection (low threshold in those with bronchiectasis and cystic fibrosis).
- Consider oral tranexamic acid (15–25 mg/kg tds, max. 1 g tds).
- CT chest ± bronchoscopy and further investigations as appropriate.

Massive haemoptysis (100–600 ml in 24 hours)
- Manage as above.
- High-flow oxygen.
- IV crystalloids.
- If known which lung the blood is coming from (such as post bronchoscopy or instrumentation) then nurse patient with bleeding lung down.
- Adrenaline nebulizer (5 ml of 1:1000).
- Bronchoscopy is rarely useful in the acute massive bleed. Fibreoptic bronchoscopy has no role; occasionally rigid bronchoscopy (usually performed by thoracic surgeons) will allow clot removal/diathermy/ haemostasis with thrombin glue/iced saline or vasoconstrictor lavage/tamponade of bleeding using a Fogarty catheter.
- Selective bronchial angiography and embolization. Tertiary service. Source of bleeding difficult to determine but dilated tortuous vessels embolized (>2.5 mm). Spinal artery thombosis potential complication.

- IV vasopressin (20 units in 100 ml 5% dextrose given over 15 minutes followed by an infusion 0.2 units/min for 36 hours) or terlipressin (2 mg stat then 1–2 mg every 4–6 hours), which has fewer side effects, is sometimes useful until bleeding is settles.
- Urgent referral to ITU may be required. Consider intubation with double-lumen tube.
- Lobectomy may be considered as a last resort.

In palliative cases with massive haemoptysis the above management may not be appropriate. Use high-flow oxygen and consider diamorphine to alleviate distressing symptoms.

Chest pain

☼ Chest pain

There are many causes of chest pain, both respiratory and non-respiratory. Differentiating between them relies on a thorough history and examination, giving rise to diagnosis by pattern recognition, as well as appropriate investigations.

Causes

Respiratory

Lung parenchyma

- Pneumonia: associated with fever, rigors, sputum production. Consolidation on CXR.
- Malignancy: either associated with a complication such as infection, effusion, or PE, or due to invasion of chest wall.
- Sarcoid: cough and SOB. Review skin, joint, or eye problems.

Pleura

- Pneumothorax: sudden-onset pleuritic pain and SOB. Young tall male smokers at increased risk of primary spontaneous pneumothorax.
- Pleural effusion.
- Pleurisy: consider viral, drug-induced, SLE, familial Mediterranean fever.

Pulmonary vasculature

- Pulmonary embolus: pleuritic pain, SOB, haemoptysis, and risk factors (particularly pregnancy). PIOPED study found 97% presented with pain, SOB, or tachycardia, with 90% presenting with SOB, tachycardia, or DVT.

Cardiac

- Ischaemic heart disease: classic story. Worse on exertion/relieved with rest, radiates to jaw/arm. Associated with sweating, nausea, SOB. Cardiac risk factors.
- Aortic dissection: sudden severe ripping pain. More common in older men. Risk factors include hypertension and less commonly Marfan's syndrome, aortic coarctation, and rarely pregnancy. Check pulses, asymmetrical BP readings in arms, murmur of aortic regurgitation, ischaemic ECG, widened mediastinum on CXR.
- Pericarditis: pain reduced on sitting forward. Listen for rub. ECG: widespread ST elevation.
- Valvular heart disease: particularly aortic stenosis. Progressive angina, dyspnoea, and syncope.

Gastro-intestinal

- Gastro-oesophageal reflux: burning pain, radiates to back and jaw. Worse after meals or on lying. ?Relieved by antacids.
- Mediastinitis: Boerhaeve's syndrome (oesophageal rupture after vomiting), iatrogenic, caustic ingestion, and Barrett's oesophagus. Air in mediastinum on CXR. Septic.
- Pancreatitis/biliary.
- PUD.

Chest wall
- Musculoskeletal: insidious, long history, associated trauma or recent repetitive activity. Worse on movement and inspiration.
- Fractured rib.
- Costochondritis (Tietze's syndrome).
- Autoimmune disease (SLE, rheumatoid involving thoracic joints).
- Skin and sensory nerves, e.g. shingles.

History
Pain
- Nature: respiratory pain is typically pleuritic, whilst most cardiac causes of pain have characteristic patterns.
- Site.
- Severity.
- Duration.
- Radiation.
- Exacerbating or relieving factors (e.g. pain associated with pericarditis eases with leaning forward).
- Similar pain in past.

Other features
- Associated symptoms: cough, fever, sputum production, haemoptysis, SOB, nausea, sweating.
- Risk factors: recent travel, immobility, trauma, cardiac risk factors.
- Past medical history and family history.

Examination
- Observations: temperature, oxygen saturations, heart rate, blood pressure, respiratory rate.
- Chest wall tenderness does not exclude an underlying cause of chest pain.
- Examine for associated features of disease:
  - Rashes, ulcers, arthritis in autoimmune conditions.
  - Clubbing, cachexia, and lymphadenopathy in lung cancer.
- Auscultation and percussion of chest.
- Listen for pericardial rubs.
- Examine abdomen.

Investigations
- FBC.
- U&Es (severity scoring in pneumonia).
- LFTs and amylase if concerns re GI pathology.
- Inflammatory markers.
- D-dimer: if low or intermediate suspicion of PE (high negative predictive value).
- Troponin at 12 hours if suspect cardiac pain.
- ECG.
- CXR.
- ABG (if oxygen saturations <92%).

Further investigations as appropriate
- V/Q or CTPA if D-dimer positive, no alternative diagnosis more likely, or high clinical suspicion of PE (📖 p. 184 *PE algorithm*).
- ECHO for investigation of cardiac causes.
- Diagnostic pleural tap.
- Serum autoantibodies.
- CT chest.
- Bone scan.

Respiratory failure

☼ Acute hypoxaemic respiratory failure

Type 1 respiratory failure occurs in the presence of a pO_2 <8kPa with a normal or low pCO_2. This is most commonly caused by a ventilation–perfusion mismatch at the alveolar level, with an increase in the alveolar–arterial (A–a) gradient (see below). It is hard to differentiate between acute and chronic hypoxemic respiratory failure on blood gases alone; other markers such as polycythaemia and cor pulmonale point to chronicity.

Causes of acute type 1 respiratory failure

Pulmonary
- Asthma.
- Pneumonia.
- Pneumothorax.
- Exacerbation of pre-existing pulmonary disease (COPD, bronchiectasis, interstitial lung disease).
- Pulmonary haemorrhage.

Vascular
- Pulmonary embolism.
- Cardiogenic pulmonary oedema.
- Intra-cardiac shunt.
- AV malformation in the lung.
- Pulmonary arterial hypertension.

Upper airway
- Acute epiglottitis.
- Tumour or foreign body.

Pathophysiology

Acute hypoxaemic respiratory failure occurs in the presence of a ventilation–perfusion mismatch or shunting. With a mismatch, areas of underventilated lung which are still adequately perfused cause hypoxaemia, whilst in shunting, either intrapulmonary or intracardiac, mixed venous blood bypasses ventilated lung. In both cases the A–a oxygen difference (usually <2 kPa) is increased. An increase in the A–a oxygen gradient indicates pulmonary disease to be the cause of hypoxia.

$$A–a \text{ gradient} = PaO_2 - (PaO_2 + PaCO_2/0.8)$$

where A indicates alveolar (% inspired oxygen of 100 − 7, i.e. if breathing air 21% of (100 − 7) ≈ 20 kPa), a indicates arterial, and 0.8 is the respiratory quotient (⌷ Chapter 53 for more detailed explanation).

Even in the normal lung, not all alveoli are optimally perfused and ventilated. In general the apices are relatively underperfused compared with the bases because of the effects of gravity on pulmonary blood flow.

Alveoli that are optimally perfused but not adequately ventilated are called low V/Q units and act like a shunt. Low V/Q units may occur because of either underventilation secondary to a pathological process in the airway or interstitium or relative overperfusion, such as in pulmonary embolism, with diversion of blood away from the parts of the lung where flow is obstructed by emboli.

A shunt is present where hypoxia cannot be corrected despite the administration of 100% inhaled oxygen. Pulmonary shunts occur in the presence of pneumonia, atelectasis, and severe pulmonary oedema, whilst vascular shunts occur in atrial and ventricular septal defects, patent ductus arteriosis or foramen ovale, or an arteriovenous malformation in the lung.

Clinical assessment

History

- Features of infection such as cough, fever, sputum production, or pleuritic chest pain. Possibility of aspiration.
- PMH of cardiac or valvular disease. History of chest pain, increasing shortness of breath on exertion, or orthopnoea and paroxysmal nocturnal dyspnoea.
- Unilateral leg swelling; history of immobility or recent surgery. Previous thromboembolism.
- Known pulmonary disease.
- Drug history (particularly possible pulmonary toxic drugs), environmental exposure.

Examination

On observation the patient is likely to be dyspnoeic and may be cyanosed. Evidence of cor pulmonale may point to chronicity. Stridor indicates an upper respiratory airway problem, whilst audible wheeze is suggestive of asthma or COPD.

Examine for valvular heart disease and percuss/auscultate chest to exclude effusion, pneumothorax, or consolidation. Look for peripheral oedema, calf swelling, and signs of associated disease such as clubbing, rheumatoid joints, and skin rashes.

Investigation

- FBC to investigate for polycythaemia. U&Es, cardiac enzymes.
- CXR.
- ABG.
- ECG – acute right heart strain is suggestive of large pulmonary embolus.
- Further investigation as appropriate:
  - Pulmonary function testing.
  - CT chest.
  - ECHO.
  - Autoimmune screen.
  - Angiography.

Management

- Ensure airway is patent and safe.
  - If stridor is present seek an urgent ENT opinion and consider use of Heliox as interim measure if required (📖 Chapter 45).
  - Intubate if concerns.

- Correct hypoxaemia with high-flow oxygen. Aim to maintain oxygen saturations >92%. If hypoxaemia cannot be corrected with oxygen alone then consider CPAP if appropriate, or intubation and ventilation.
- Discuss with ITU, particularly if requiring high-percentage oxygen or non-invasive ventilation to maintain oxygen levels.
- Treat underlying cause.

☼ Acute hypercapnic respiratory failure

Type 2 respiratory failure occurs when there is a low PaO_2 (<8 kPa) in the presence of a raised CO_2 level (>6kPa). Hypercapnic respiratory failure is the end result of many causes of respiratory failure (e.g. pneumonia, pulmonary oedema), not just chronic lung conditions such as COPD. It results from an overall reduction is ventilation (alveolar hypoventilation), an increase in the proportion of dead-space ventilation, or an imbalance between load and capacity.

Causes

Reduction in minute ventilation
- Neuromuscular disorders affecting the respiratory muscles, such as muscular dystrophy, myasthenia gravis, polio, and Guillain–Barré syndrome.
- CNS depression
  - Drug overdose.
  - Vascular abnormality or tumour affecting the brainstem.
  - Hypothyroidism.
- Chest wall abnormalities (such as severe kyphoscoliosis).
- Morbid obesity (causing obesity hypoventilation syndrome).

Increased dead-space ventilation
- Obstructive airways disease, such as COPD, asthma, and cystic fibrosis.
- Upper airway causes such as tracheal tumours and epiglottitis.

Alveolar abnormalities
Hypercapnia may also occur in cases of hypoxaemic respiratory failure where diffuse alveolar filling initially causes shunting and increased work of breathing; however, with time this may lead to decreased alveolar ventilation. Examples of this include severe pulmonary oedema, pneumonia and pulmonary haemorrhage.

Acute versus chronic
This can be determined from the blood gases. In acute conditions, e.g. asthma and pneumonia, hypercapnia will be associated with acidosis and a normal bicarbonate. In conditions with chronic hypercapnia, the bicarbonate will be raised because of renal compensation. Acidosis may or may not be present depending on the degree of acute respiratory compromise.

Other factors that suggest chronicity include evidence of right heart strain and cor pulmonale.

Assessment

- Full history including;
  - Prior chest problems.
  - Muscle weakness, swallowing difficulties, change in speech.
  - Breathlessness on lying flat or swimming (suggestive of diaphragmatic paralysis).
  - Drug history.
- Examine for evidence of associated pathology;
  - Chest wall abnormalities such as kyphosis or scoliosis.
  - Muscle wasting or fasciculation.
  - Signs of hyperinflation/prolonged expiratory phase (obstructive airways disease).
  - Features of drug overdose such as pinpoint pupils with opiates.
  - Paradoxical abdominal movement on breathing.

Investigations

- Routine bloods to include TFTs.
- CXR.
- ABG.
- ECG (for evidence of right heart strain).
- Lung function tests, including where necessary;
  - Lying and standing VC if concerns regarding neuromuscular involvement.
  - SNIP (inspiratory pressure) to investigate diaphragmatic weakness).

Respiratory failure is uncommon in obstructive disease where FEV_1 >1 L.

Further management

- First ensure a safe airway and check breathing and circulation.
- Establish IV access.
- Commence treatment for underlying cause, e.g. nebulized bronchodilators, diuretics.
- Ongoing management will depend on cause of hypercapnia.
  - *Acute condition*, e.g. asthma, pneumonia: discussion with ITU for consideration of ventilation (if appropriate).
  - *Chronic condition*, e.g. COPD/neuromuscular disease: controlled oxygen, monitoring CO_2. May need NIV or invasive ventilation (📖 Chapter 47).

ⓘ Cor pulmonale

Cor pulmonale describes the cardiovascular consequences of chronic hypoxia resulting from chronic lung disease, usually referring to a combination of pulmonary hypertension and fluid retention. Chronic hypoxaemia, often in association with hypercapnia, results in progressive pulmonary hypertension and right ventricular remodelling (hypertrophy and dilatation). Although right ventricular output is often maintained, right ventricular failure may occur over time.

Diagnosis

- Chronic hypoxic lung disease (+ hypercapnia usually).
- Pulmonary hypertension.
- Fluid retention.

Pulmonary hypertension

Pulmonary hypertension (defined in cor pulmonale as a resting pulmonary artery pressure (PAP) >20 mmHg) is thought to arise as a result of pulmonary vascular bed remodelling in response to chronic alveolar hypoxia (distinct from acute vasoconstriction secondary to acute hypoxia). Associated hypercapnic acidosis and polycythaemia (secondary to hypoxia) may also contribute to increased pulmonary pressures.

Fluid retention

Fluid retention is not usually the result of right heart failure *per se* (as cardiac output in cor pulmonale is maintained), but rather occurs through renal retention of salt and water in a neurohormonal response to hypoxaemia. Thus peripheral oedema may arise in the absence of a truly 'failing' right ventricle, as capillary permeability increases in response to the associated hypercapnic state.

Causes

Three major groups of respiratory disease cause cor pulmonale; the majority (estimated around 80%) are due to obstructive lung disease. The following list excludes pulmonary vascular disease (primary pulmonary hypertension, chronic thrombo-emboli, veno-occlusive disease). Asterisks indicate more common causes.

Obstructive lung disease

- Chronic obstructive pulmonary disease.*
- Asthma (+ irreversible airways obstruction).
- Bronchiectasis.
- Cystic fibrosis.
- Obliterative bronchiolitis.

Restrictive lung disease

- Kyphoscoliosis.*
- Idiopathic pulmonary fibrosis.
- Neuromuscular disease (myopathies, diaphragm paralysis).
- Post pulmonary TB (fibrosis, pleural thickening, thoracoplasty).
- Pneumoconioses.
- Drug-induced lung fibrosis.
- Fibrotic extrinsic allergic alveolitis.
- Fibrosis secondary to connective tissue disease.

Breathing pattern dysfunction

- Obstructive sleep apnoea.*
- Obesity hypoventilation* ('Pickwickian syndrome').
- Any cause of chronic 'central' hypoventilation (syringobulbia, brainstem pathology, etc).

Clinical features

The incidence of cor pulmonale is unknown, although studies have suggested a prevalence of 0.3% in patients with chronic respiratory disease and hypoxia. Patients generally have a PaO_2 <8 kPa on air and are known to have chronic lung disease, although they may present *de novo* with cor pulmonale.

There is controversy over whether peripheral oedema and raised JVP are the result of true right heart failure or simply fluid (and salt) retention in response to renal hypoxia.

Patients may present with features of cor pulmonale during an acute exacerbation of underlying lung disease.

History

Assuming a *de novo* presentation of cor pulmonale, enquire about:
- Features of chronic lung disease. Specifically:
  - Progressive dyspnoea.
  - Smoking history.
  - Childhood respiratory disease (including asthma).
  - Sleep history (Ⓜ Chapter 41).
  - Sputum production.
  - Previous TB (including surgical treatment).
  - Occupational history.
  - Drug history.
- Muscle weakness/swallowing difficulties.
- Fragmented sleep pattern, early morning headaches/confusion.
- Skeletal abnormalities.
- Symptoms of connective tissue disease.

Examination

Features specific to cor pulmonale.
- Signs of hypoxia (cyanosis, plethora secondary to polycythaemia).
- Signs of hypercapnia (asterixis, conjunctival suffusion, bounding pulse, vasodilatation, confusion).
- Raised JVP.
- Ankle/dependent oedema.
- Ascites.
- Signs of pulmonary hypertension (right ventricular heave, loud P2).
- Signs of tricuspid regurgitation (pansystolic murmur, V waves in the JVP) caused by dilatation of the RV (functional TR).

Also assess for features of possible causes (see individual chapters) as follows.
- Hyperinflation/wheeze (obstructive airways disease).
- Crackles/clubbing/poor expansion (fibrosis/restriction).
- Thoracic cage abnormalities (including surgery).
- Diaphragm weakness (abdominal indrawing on inspiration).
- Evidence of myopathy.
- Neck size.
- Evidence of connective tissue disease.

Investigations

The aim is to establish the cause of cor pulmonale.
- Pulse oximetry: cor pulmonale is unlikely if SaO_2 >92%.
- ECG: evidence of right heart strain (P pulmonale, right axis deviation, right bundle branch block).
- FBC: polycythaemia common in chronic hypoxaemia.
- ABGs: expect hypoxia and hypercapnia.
- CXR: bulky pulmonary arteries, changes consistent with underlying lung disease.
- Pulmonary function tests: obstruction/restriction.
- Echocardiography: RV structure and function, presence of tricuspid regurgitation, estimation of PAP (only if TR present).
- Overnight oximetry or sleep study.
- Nerve conduction studies/EMG.
- Tests for specific conditions (e.g. Acetylcholine receptor antibodies in myasthenia) or MRI of brain.

Management

1. Treat underlying disorder

Optimize management of the underlying disease (e.g. bronchodilators, steroid therapy, CPAP).

2. Supplemental oxygen

Reversing alveolar hypoxia may prevent further increases in PAP. Caution is needed as many patients are hypercapnic, and a careful assessment is required to ensure that patients do not 'retain' CO_2 on oxygen therapy (i.e. loss of hypoxic drive). Long-term oxygen therapy (>15 hours/day) is generally required, extrapolating from two trials in COPD demonstrating improved survival on oxygen therapy.

3. Non-invasive ventilation

Long-term overnight NIV is useful in cases of hypoventilation. Acute NIV is not required in patients with cor pulmonale unless given for acute hypercapnic and acidotic respiratory failure.

4. Diuretic therapy for peripheral oedema

Diuretics are used to prevent uncomfortable peripheral oedema. However, diuresis does not affect the underlying disease process and may exacerbate the problem (decreased filling pressure to the right ventricle). Some remaining ankle oedema is acceptable and likely, and over-use of diuretic to treat this problem is not recommended.

Prognosis

Prolonged survival (>10 years) can be seen after the first episode of peripheral oedema secondary to cor pulmonale. However, a higher level of pulmonary artery hypertension has been associated with poorer prognosis in COPD.

Common chest radiograph presentations

! **Unilateral lucency on the CXR**

Increased transradiancy of one area of the CXR or one hemithorax compared with the other. The most common cause is technical factors (e.g. rotation). This can usually be identified by comparing the degree of lucency of the soft tissues on each side.

Differential diagnosis

Pneumothorax

- Look for the thin shadow of the lung edge (visceral pleura) which should be visible in incomplete pneumothorax (Chapter 58).
- Look for complete absence of lung markings lateral to this.
- Blunting of the costophrenic angle is commonly present (small associated pleural effusion).
- Complete pneumothorax: look for mediastinal shift away from the affected side.
- If mediastinal shift is marked (especially if hemidiaphragm is depressed) consider tension pneumothorax (Chapter 58).
- Tension pneumothorax should be diagnosed clinically and treated immediately without a CXR.

Lung hyper-expansion

Causes

- Previous lobectomy.
- Ipsilateral collapse.
- Asymmetrical emphysema.
- Air trapping secondary to foreign body.

Bullae

These are abnormally dilated air spaces within the lung as a result of emphysematous change, usually occurring in the upper lobes. Although usually small, they may occupy one-third of a hemithorax. Their importance is that they may be mistaken for a pneumothorax in an acutely dyspnoeic patient with COPD. The round rim of a bullus may be visible and faint lung markings may differentiate them from pneumothorax. Thoracic CT is often required to be certain.

Chest wall abnormality

Decrease in the tissues overlying the lung may result in increased transradiancy. The most common cause is mastectomy, but it may also occur with congenital absence of pectoralis major (Poland's syndrome).

Pulmonary embolus

Uncommonly pulmonary embolus may be associated with oligaemic vascular markings in the affected area of the lung (Westermark's sign).

Approach to the patient

History

- Sudden onset shortness of breath (pneumothorax, rarely PE).
- Acute chest pain (pneumothorax, PE).
- A history of COPD or long-term smoking (emphysema, bullae).
- A history of foreign body inhalation.
- Previous surgery (lobectomy, mastectomy).
- Weight loss, haemoptysis, bone pain (obstructing bronchial carcinoma, collapse).
- Symptoms of chronic infection (TB lymphadenopathy).

Examination

- Tracheal shift (pneumothorax, collapse).
- Hyper-resonant percussion + absent/decreased breath sounds (pneumothorax, bulla).
- Above + unwell patient (hypotension, profound tracheal shift): consider tension pneumothorax.
- Surgical scars (thoracotomy, mastectomy).
- Signs of obstructive lung disease (pneumothorax, bulla).
- Cachexia, lymphadenopathy (malignancy, TB).
- Check for expansion of the contralateral lung: if this is reduced, suggests this is the abnormal lung (i.e. the lung that appears lucent is in fact normal whilst the 'normal' lung has increased shadowing).

Investigations

Guided by likely diagnosis on the basis of above.

Key points

- In tension pneumothorax, no investigations (not even a CXR) should be conducted until tension has been relieved definitively (drain placement).
- Differentiation of pneumothorax and bullae in an acutely breathless COPD patient can be difficult: thoracic CT scan is the investigation of choice.
- Lung collapse may be subtle and missed on a CXR: thoracic CT is reliable here.
- Bronchoscopy may be required to diagnose + treat foreign body inhalation.

Management

Dependent on diagnosis.

Key points

- Tension pneumothorax requires immediate treatment.
- If there is diagnostic difficulty between pneumothorax and bullae, delay drain insertion until appropriate imaging or senior review.
- Drain insertion into a bulla can cause substantial bleeding and result in air leak which may be resistant to treatment.
- 📖 p. 169 (pneumothorax algorithm).

① Unilateral shadowing on the CXR

Unilateral shadowing on the CXR is a common clinical scenario with a wide differential diagnosis. The important features required to reach a diagnosis are as follows.

- Thorough history and examination.
- Knowledge of the differential diagnosis.
- Ability to recognize radiological patterns.
- Rapid appropriate investigations.

Abnormalities on the CXR may be chronic, and the provision of previous CXRs is invaluable to assess whether the changes are new.

Differential diagnosis

Consolidation

Also known as air-space shadowing. It is caused by opacification of air spaces within the lung. Any process which results in filling (usually by fluid) of the alveoli and small airways will result in consolidation. Most patients with consolidation will be breathless and may be hypoxic (V/Q mismatch in consolidated lung).

Radiological appearance

- Ill defined shadowing with obscured vascular markings.
- Air bronchograms are pathogneumonic (air filled bronchi contrasting against fluid-filled underlying lung).
- Usually sharply demarcated if adjacent to the pleural or interlobar fissures (☐ Chapter 58).

The differential diagnosis is wide, and only relevant acute causes are covered here.

Common

- Infection (bacterial, viral).
- Infarction.
- Cardiogenic pulmonary oedema (usually bilateral).
- Non-cardiogenic pulmonary oedema (usually bilateral).

Less common

- Drug reactions.
- Haemorrhage.
- Malignancy (lymphoma, bronchoalveolar cell carcinoma).
- Cryptogenic organizing pneumonia.
- Sarcoidosis.

Pleural effusion

Fluid accumulation between the visceral and parietal pleura. ☐ Chapter 24 for causes and details on investigation.

Radiological appearance

- Around 200 ml of fluid needs to be present before visible on a PA CXR. Initially blunting of costophrenic angle (☐ Chapter 58).
- Normal appearance is of opacity obscuring hemidiaphragm with presence of a meniscus.

- If massive, may cause 'lung white-out': look for mediastinal shift away from effusion.
- Diffuse hazy shadowing throughout hemithorax in supine films.

Collapse

Partial or complete volume loss from a lung or lobe, also called atelectasis. May occur in areas of a single lobe, multiple lobes, or an entire lung.

Radiological appearance

Look for:
- Volume loss
  - Displaced fissure.
  - Loss of aeration.
  - Crowded bronchi/vessels.
- Compensation for volume loss
  - Elevated hemi-diaphragm.
  - Displaced hilum/trachea.
  - Rib crowding.
  - Hyperinflation of non-involved lung.

Differential diagnosis

- Bronchial tumour.
- Enlarged lymph nodes (malignancy, TB, sarcoid).
- Viscid secretions (includes infection, post-anaesthesia).
- Pulmonary embolus (plate like atelectasis).
- Diaphragmatic weakness/paralysis (lower atelectasis).

Infarction

A rare result of pulmonary embolic disease, resulting in peripheral wedge-shaped opacities. Usually lower lobes.

Approach to the patient with unilateral CXR shadowing

History

- Symptoms of infection (infective consolidation/effusion).
- Dyspnoea (speed of onset important).
- Chest pain (PE, pleural effusion, consolidation abutting pleura).
- Symptoms and risk factors for heart failure.
- Risk score for embolic disease.
- Systemic symptoms (malignancy, TB, sarcoid).
- Smoking history.
- Drug history.
- Occupational history (pleural disease).
- Pre-existing lung disease.
- Previous surgery (atelectasis, pneumonectomy).

Examination

- Thoracotomy scar.
- 'Classical' signs of consolidation (increased breath sounds, bronchial breathing ± crackles, increased vocal resonance, whispering pectoriloquy).
- Signs of effusion (stony dull percussion, decreased breath sounds, tracheal shift away if large, decreased vocal resonance).

- Paradoxical abdominal movement (diaphragm paralysis).
- Cachexia, lymphadenopathy (TB, malignancy).

Investigations

Vary depending on likely diagnosis.

Key points

- Thoracic CT valuable if diagnostic doubt (e.g.?collapse/?consolidation).
- Thoracic ultrasound valuable to rapidly exclude effusion.
- Pleural aspiration should be delayed until further imaging if any diagnostic doubt or failed first attempt ('dry tap').
- Bronchoscopy may be used to diagnose cause of collapse.

Management

See individual sections for detailed management of each condition.

! Bilateral pulmonary infiltrates on the CXR

Bilateral non-confluent airspace and interstitial shadowing is a frequent and often challenging clinical scenario. The cause may be obvious; however sometimes it is not and a thorough review of history, examination, investigations, and medications is needed. Considering the differential diagnoses in the immunocompetent and immunocompromised separately provides a structure to begin the initial assessment.

Causes in immunocompetent patients

- Infection.
  - Bacterial infection.
  - Tuberculous infection.
  - Viral infection.
  - Fungal infection, including PCP.
- Alveolar haemorrhage.
  - Wegener's granulomatosis.
  - Microscopic polyangiitis.
  - Churg–Strauss syndrome.
  - Goodpasture's disease.
- Pulmonary oedema.
- ARDS/ALI: non-cardiogenic pulmonary oedema.
- Interstitial lung disease:
  - Sarcoidosis.
  - UIP/NSIP/LIP/DIP/RBILD.
  - AIP: idiopathic ARDS.
  - Cryptogenic organizing pneumonia (COP).
- Drug-induced lung disease, including illicit drug use.
- Eosinophilic pneumonia.
- Malignant disease.
  - Alveolar cell carcinoma.
  - Lymphoma.
  - Lymphangitis carcinomatosis.

- Hypersensitivity pneumonitis.
- ABPA.

Causes of predominantly upper lobe infiltrates
- Sarcoidosis (and berylliosis).
- Tuberculosis.
- Radiation therapy (may be unilateral).
- Hypersensitivity pneumonitis.
- Ankylosing spondylitis.

Causes in the immunocompromised patient

In modern medical practice, patients are frequently immunocompromised (Chapter 13 for detailed discussion). Causes include cytotoxic chemotherapy, malignancy, immunosuppressive therapy for non-malignant conditions, or post-transplant and congenital or acquired immuno-deficiencies.

Such patients commonly present with acute respiratory symptoms. All the conditions which can occur in the immunocompetent individual can also occur in the immunocompromised. Infection remains the largest cause.

The differential diagnosis of bilateral pulmonary infiltrates in the immunocompromised includes the following.
- Infection.
  - Bacterial: different spectrum of organisms, including rare bacteria e.g. *Nocardia*.
  - Viral: CMV pneumonitis, varicella.
  - Fungus: *Aspergillus*, PCP, *Candida*, *Cryptococcus*.
  - TB and non-tuberculous mycobacteria.
- Alveolar haemorrhage.
- Pulmonary oedema.
- ARDS/ALI: non-cardiogenic pulmonary oedema:
  - TRALI: transfusion associated ALI may complicate patients requiring large blood transfusions.
- Drug-induced lung disease: many chemotherapy agents are associated with interstitial lung disease.
- Malignant disease.
  - Alveolar cell carcinoma.
  - Lymphoma.
  - Lymphangitis carcinomatosis.
  - Post-transplant lymphoproliferative disease.
- Interstitial lung disease:
  - COP.
  - NSIP/LIP/DIP.
- Graft versus host disease.

Part 2

Clinical scenarios

Inhalational injury

☼ Smoke inhalation

The approach to a patient who has suffered from significant smoke inhalation follows the basic airway, breathing, circulation concept. Remember to ask for details about the incident as other chemicals may have been inhaled in the smoke (see hazardous chemicals below).

The damage caused by smoke inhalation causes the following levels of injury.

Upper airways
- Laryngeal oedema.
- Mucosal inflammation.
- Ciliary dysfunction.

Lower airways
- Bronchospasm.
- Bronchial oedema/mucosal inflammation.
- Ciliary dysfunction.
- Reduced surfactant.
- Systemic inflammatory response.

Symptoms
- Hoarse voice.
- Difficulty breathing/breathlessness.
- Retrosternal chest pain.

Signs
Airway
- Look for:
  - loss of eyebrows.
  - burnt nasal hair.
  - facial burns, particularly around the nose or mouth.
  - oropharyngeal burns.
- Carbonaceous sputum.
- Stridor.
- Laryngeal oedema.

Breathing
- Tachypnoea (RR > 24).
- Inspiratory crackles, wheeze, or stridor.
- Low oxygen saturations.
⚠ Saturations remain high in the presence of COHb (see carbon monoxide poisoning below).

Circulation
- Tachycardia.
- Hypotension may be present if there are large area burns to the skin or in the presence of ARDS.

Investigations
- CXR (may show pulmonary infiltrates).
- ABG.
- Measure COHb.

Management

- Early intubation in the presence of laryngeal oedema or airway burns. This may be a difficult intubation or require a surgical airway (📖 Chapter 42).
- If ventilated consider a 'lung protective' ventilatory strategy (permissive hypercapnia with low pressure/volume).
- High-flow oxygen.
- IV fluid replacement.
- Close observation for signs of ARDS.
- Steroid use and prophylactic antibiotics are areas where opinion varies on their effectiveness. Cilia and mucosal damage makes infection more likely.

✚ Hazardous chemicals

Hazardous chemicals are used in manufacturing and the public may be exposed through accidental spills, explosions, and fires. In modern society, non-accidental release of hazardous chemicals can occur in situations associated with military use and acts of terrorism.

The effect of each chemical varies, depending upon its solubility, the mechanism by which it causes damage, systemic effects, and characteristics of the exposure. Highly soluble substances are less likely to reach the lung parenchyma.

Chemicals can produce direct cellular damage (e.g. alkalis and acids), mucous secretion, form oxygen free radicals which in turn cause damage (e.g. oxides of nitrogen), or stimulate parasympathetic receptors and trigger smooth muscle bronchoconstriction (inducing airway hyper-reactivity and bronchospasm).

Damage to nasal passages and oro-pharynx can cause

- Oedema.
- Ulceration.
- Haemorrhage.

Damage to the trachea and bronchi can cause

- paralysis of the cilia.
- increased mucous production.
- mucosal oedema.
- Exudates.
- submucosal haemorrhage.
- formation of pseudomembranes.

This can result in

- bronchiolitis.
- obliterative bronchiolitis.
- organizing pneumonia.

Damage to the alveoli and interstitium can cause
- epithelial necrosis.
- Sloughing.
- formation of hyaline membranes.
- alveolar capillary leakage leading to ARDS.

In the long term this can result in permanent interstitial fibrosis

⚠ Patients may still have chemical contamination both as a contact hazard and a vapor hazard. Proper precautions must be taken to avoid medical staff becoming casualties.

Management
- Assess for upper airway obstruction
  - Look for stridor, drooling, tracheal tug.
  - Oedema, mucosal sloughing, haemorrhage.
  - Consider intubation/tracheostomy early.
- ABG.
- Assess for COHb.
- CXR (may be unhelpful early on).
- ECG.
- Supplemental oxygen (high levels may increase oxidative damage).
- Bronchodilators.
- Fluid replacement (avoid contributing to pulmonary oedema but essential in ARDS).
- Consider specific antidotes if nature of chemical exposure known.
- Steroids and prophylactic antibiotics: efficacy not clear; some advocate their use.

Table 10.1 Chemical effects

Inhalant	Sources	Mechanism/injury	Treatment
Asphyxiants			
Hydrogen cyanide	Chemical warfare, burning polyurethane	Inhibits cytochrome oxidase activity, inhibiting ATP production	Sodium thiosulphate, sodium nitrite, dicobalt edentate, hydroxocobalamin
Hydrogen sulphide	Metallurgy, chemical manufacture, water treatment, volcanic gases	Inhibits cytochrome oxidase activity, inhibiting ATP production	Supportive
Carbon monoxide	Gas heaters, smoke inhalation, miners	Competes with O_2 for Hb binding sites	High-flow O_2, hyperbaric O_2
Irritant gases			
Phosgene, isocyanates	Chemical warfare, chemical and dye manufacture	Necrosis of tracheal to bronchiolar mucosa, oedema, haemorrhage, ARDS	Supportive
Ammonia	Agriculture, plastics, dyes	Irritation of mucous membranes, upper airway oedema and obstruction	Supportive
Chlorine	Household cleaners, textiles, sewage treatment, swimming pools	Liberates hydrogen chloride and O_2 free radicals. Pulmonary oedema, tracheobronchitis	Supportive
Sulphur dioxide	Smelting, paper and chemical manufacture	Pharyngeal and pulmonary oedema. Obliterative bronchiolitis	Supportive Systemic corticosteroids may benefit
Nitrogen oxides	Welders, dye manufacture, silo fillers, explosives use	Potent oxidizers > tissue inflammation + impair surfactant. Also causes metHb. Pneumonitis, bronchiolitis, pulmonary oedema	Supportive Systemic corticosteroids may benefit
Vesicant			
Mustard gas, Lewisite	Chemical warfare	Chemical pneumonitis, pulmonary oedema, pseudomembrane formation	Supportive Dimercaprol for Lewisite

Table 10.1 (Contd.)

Inhalant	Sources	Mechanism/injury	Treatment
Systemic toxins			
Nerve agents (Tabun, sarin, soman, ricin, VX)	Chemical warfare	Anticholinesterase effect against acetylcholinesterase. Causes meiosis, glandular secretion, bradycardia, AV block, fasciculation, paralysis, seizures, respiratory depression	Atropine, oximes (e.g. pralidoxime), benzodiazepines
Metals/metal compounds			
Cadmium	Fertilizers	Pneumonitis. Long-term causes emphysema	Supportive
Cobalt	Phosphate fertilizers	Wheezing, pneumonitis, asthma	Bronchodilators
Zinc	Zinc mining, steel manufacturing	Dyspnoea, flu-like illness	Supportive
Welding fumes	Welding	Airways obstruction	Bronchodilators
Beryllium	Limited industrial use	Pneumonitis, tracheitis. Chronic response is berylliosis (sarcoid-like)	Supportive

⚙ Carbon monoxide

⚠ Cyanosis does not occur with CO poisoning. Pulse oximetry gives false readings as COHb light absorption is similar to oxyhaemoglobin. Measure COHb if suspected.

Carbon monoxide has a 250 times greater affinity for haemoglobin than oxygen. It is not irreversibly bound and so high inspired O_2 concentrations will displace the CO from Hb. The half-life of COHb in air is 4 hours; with 100% O_2 it decreases to 40 minutes and with hyperbaric O_2 to 20 minutes.

Carbon monoxide poisoning is caused by incomplete combustion. Poorly maintained gas fires, self-poisoning, and being trapped in a burning building are the most common causes.

Clinical features
Acute
- Dyspnoea
- Fatigue
- Headaches
- Tiredness
- Tinnitus
- Tachypnoea
- Tachycardia.

If severe:
- Pulmonary oedema
- Myocardial ischaemia
- Arrhythmias
- Seizures
- Coma.

Late
- Cognitive deficits
- Focal neurology
- Personality change.

Investigations
- Remember that pulse oximetry and arterial PaO_2 may appear normal.
- Measure COHb (breath analyser, arterial or venous sample);
    - Normal COHb levels <4% in non-smokers, ~10% in heavy smokers.
    - >20% COHb (>10% in children) is significant CO poisoning.
    - >30% COHb confusion.
    - >35% COHb coma.
    - >50% COHb death.
- ECG.
- CXR.
- Cardiac monitor.

Management
- Give high-concentration (100%) O_2.
- If consciousness is impaired, intubate and ventilate.
- Consider hyperbaric O_2, particularly if COHb >20% or coma, as this displaces CO more rapidly (although it needs to be done early).
- Treat seizures.

Inhaled foreign bodies

:⚙: Inhaled foreign bodies

Everything from peas to bicycle tyre caps can make their way into the bronchial tree if circumstances allow! Lodging of a foreign body in the trachea is rare, and so this section only deals briefly with *tracheal* obstruction (🕮 Chapter 42 for more details).

Relevant anatomy

The right main bronchus is more vertical than the left in relation to the trachea, and so an aspirated foreign body will usually (but not always) end up in the right bronchial tree, most commonly the bronchus intermedius (leading to the right middle and lower lobes) or the right lower lobe.

Presentation

▶▶ *Acute airway obstruction*

- History of foreign body inhalation or choking.
- Conscious patient looking panic-stricken and pointing to mouth or throat. Ask if they are choking; they will nod.
- Silent breathing (i.e. not breathing).
- Paradoxical breathing pattern (seesaw breathing).
- Attempt the Heimlich manoeuvre (subdiaphragmatic pressure). For a conscious person, position yourself behind them, placing a fist, thumb side in, just above the navel. Grab the fist tightly with your other hand and pull abruptly upward and inward to increase airway pressure behind the obstructing object and force it from the windpipe. The procedure may need to be repeated several times before the object is dislodged.
- If anaphylaxis and associated angio-oedema, give IM adrenaline 0.5–1 mg (0.5–1 ml of 1:1000).
- ▶▶ If no improvement, call for an anaesthetist immediately, and possibly ENT surgeons.
- Apply oxygen at 10–15 L/min via reservoir bag if conscious.
- If unconscious inspect the mouth and remove any obvious obstruction.
- Leave well-fitting unbroken dentures in place.
- Attempt ventilation with self-inflating bag and mask.
- Anaesthetist to attempt intubation.
- Cricothyroidotomy may be required in desperate situations.

Non-emergency presentation

The most common situation is of acute onset of cough (more common than dyspnoea) after a clear history of aspiration or choking on a specific object.

Other symptoms include fever, haemoptysis, chest pain, wheeze, or stridor.

Much less common is the situation where the patient cannot remember aspirating and presents with a complication of chronic lobar occlusion (dyspnoea from lobar collapse, pneumonia, localized bronchiectasis, lung abscess), or simply as an incidental finding. It is not always obvious that an object has been aspirated rather than simply swallowed.

Evaluation

Plain CXR may show the offending foreign body if distinctly radio-opaque.

If complete lobar obstruction has occurred, subtle evidence of lobar/segmental collapse may be the only abnormality.

If the CXR is normal and there is a high index of suspicion, a comparison *expiratory* CXR can be helpful (shows hyperlucency/hyperinflation of lobe or lung with obstructed bronchus in comparison with remaining lung fields).

Management

Spontaneous expectoration of an inhaled foreign body can occur, but is less likely if it has nestled into a lobar or segmental bronchus.

All inhaled foreign bodies should be removed to avoid the complications described above.

The majority of patients (with no acute respiratory distress or hypoxia) can be managed as outpatients. Refer to respiratory team for prompt bronchoscopy. Retrieval of inhaled foreign bodies by fibreoptic bronchoscopy is not always possible (biopsy forceps may not manage to grasp the object firmly, although using a Dormia basket may help) and so further referral for rigid bronchoscopy (almost universally performed in UK by thoracic surgeons) may be needed. Treat concomitant infection if present.

Problems related to adverse environments

① Diving

The respiratory problems related to diving are predominantly due to the pressure changes on air within the body and gas absorption, as well as additional complications of pre-existing respiratory conditions.

The pressure changes in diving are large. Each 10 m of descent represents 100 kPa (1 atm) increase in pressure. Most problems occur on ascending from depth. The exceptions are hypothermia (which can occur at any stage) and aspiration/drowning (normally caused by equipment failure, running out of 'air', or oxygen convulsions).

Barotrauma

This is the result of trapped gas in a body cavity expanding or compressing during pressure changes in diving. The sinuses, ears, and lungs are most commonly affected. Lung compression during a breath-hold dive can result in alveolar wall rupture, haemorrhage and exudates.

During ascent, airspaces within the body expand. If ascent is rapid, this allows little time for any gas to escape the body via a normal route, resulting in an increased pressure in the gas pocket. In the ear this can rupture the tympanic membrane. In the lung this results in lung rupture with gas tracking to the mediastinum (pneumomediastinum), pulmonary vasculature (air embolism see below), and pleural space (pneumothorax).

Symptoms of pneumomediastinum and pneumothorax

Chest (central) discomfort, dyspnoea, hoarseness (pneumomediastinum).

Treatment

- Supplemental (100%) oxygen.
- Needle decompression of a pneumothorax.
- Recompression in a hyperbaric chamber.

⚠ High probability that a pneumothorax will tension. This requires urgent needle decompression.

The risk of barotrauma is reduced by making slow ascents when diving. Conditions that predispose to barotrauma and are recognized contra-indications to diving are:

- Spontaneous pneumothorax (unless bilateral surgical treatment has been performed).
- COPD (if FEV_1 <80%).
- Lung bullae or cysts.
- CF (if there is pulmonary involvement).
- Fibrotic lung disease.
- Active TB.
- Active sarcoid.

Asthma

Asthmatics may dive it they have allergic asthma but not if they have cold-, exercise-, or emotion-induced asthma.

Detailed guidelines are available from the British Thoracic Society (www.brit-thoracic.org.uk 'Diving Guidelines'). Essentially asthmatics can only dive if they are:

- Well controlled.
- Suffering no chest symptoms.
- Have not needed a therapeutic bronchodilator in the last 48 hours.
- Have normal spirometry.

For more information on medical conditions and diving, visit www.uksdmc. co.uk (UK Sport and Diving medical Committee).

Decompression illness/Caisson disease

- As pressure increases during descent, nitrogen dissolves into blood and other tissues and fluids.
- Ascent should be slow to allow time for this nitrogen to come out of solution. If this does not occur, bubbles are formed, compromising blood flow.
- This condition is termed 'the bends', referring to pain in the limbs and joints caused by micro-infarction, or 'the chokes', occurring as a result of pulmonary circulation compromise from a large number of bubbles collecting in the pulmonary capillary bed (air embolism).
- This condition is most commonly caused by a rapid ascent or by operating outside the boundaries of dive tables which indicate a safe decompression plan for a given duration and depth of dive.

Symptoms/signs

- Fatigue.
- Malaise.
- Rash.
- Limb pains ('the bends').
- Paraesthesia or numbness.
- Paralysis.
- Chest tightness, cough, dyspnoea, ↓ blood pressure ('the chokes').

A pre-existing right-to-left shunt in the heart, or an AV shunt in the pulmonary circulation, can allow crossover of an air embolism, which leads to a paradoxical arterial embolus with neurological damage.

Management

- Oxygen (reduces arterial PN_2, accelerating reabsorption of bubbles).
- Lie on left side (thought to reduce the risk of an arterial embolism).
- Recompression in a hyperbaric chamber (in-water recompression by descending to depth is not advised as this process may take several hours and requires monitoring).

① Flying

The major physiological challenges involved in flying relate to the effect of lower pressures on inspired PO_2 and the possibility of rapid pressure changes.

Cabin pressure

Commercial aircraft operate at cruising altitudes between 8000 m and 12 000 m. This is because these altitudes allow for greater fuel economy and avoid weather systems. Flying at these altitudes is not possible without supplemental oxygen and/or a pressurized environment (cabin pressure).

Most commercial aircraft maintain a cabin pressure of 75–85 kPa (equivalent to 1500–2400 m 'altitude') at a cruising altitude of 10 000 m. This is not a problem for most individuals but in those with lung disease this represents a potential problem of symptomatic hypoxia.

- Patients with chronic respiratory conditions and resting SaO_2 <92% should have in-flight oxygen.
- Patients with chronic respiratory conditions and SaO_2 92–95% should have a 'fit to fly' test, where aircraft conditions can be simulated on the ground by breathing 15% FiO_2 for 15 minutes, followed by an arterial or capillary blood gas (see www.brit-thoracic.org.uk for 'Air Travel Guidelines').

Airlines can supply additional oxygen for a flight given sufficient notice, although this may incur an extra charge.

Rapid depressurization

Sudden loss of cabin pressure will result in loss of consciousness at altitudes above 6000 m. Supplemental oxygen is necessary in this event until the aircraft can descend to a lower altitude.

Pneumothorax

- The reduction in pressure involved in an ascent during a flight will result in expansion of gas trapped in a pneumothorax. This has the potential to convert a simple pneumothorax into a tension pneumothorax.
- Radiological evidence of resolution of a pneumothorax should be obtained prior to flying.
- Historically, a 6 week interval after complete resolution of a pneumothorax was advised before flying. However, revised British Thoracic Society Air Travel Guidance in 2004, confirmed that the 6 week rule had been discarded and that a minimum delay of 1 week after full radiographic resolution was satisfactory (or 2 weeks after a traumatic pneumothorax or thoracic surgery)

The closed environment and long duration of flights means that airborne communicable diseases have the potential to spread. Individuals should not fly when they pose an infection risk to other travellers (e.g. open pulmonary TB).

① Altitude

Increasing altitude results in a number of physiological stresses. There is falling ambient temperature and a reduction in atmospheric pressure with increased altitude. It is also responsible for a number of acute medical problems.

Physiology

Reduced pressure decreases inspired gas PaO_2 and hence reduces tissue availability of oxygen. Given that the fractional oxygen concentration remains constant (0.21), as does the saturated vapour pressure of water at body temperature (6.3 kPa), the inspired gas PaO_2 for a given barometric pressure can be calculated as follows:

inspired gas PO_2 = 0.21 × (barometric pressure − 6.3) kPa

Table 12.1 shows the pressures for varying altitudes and equivalent inspired PaO_2. It is clear that high altitudes result in significant hypoxia from the reduction in inspired PaO_2.

Falling alveolar PO_2 results in a short-lived (<30 minutes) period of hyperventilation. This period is limited by hypocapnia (reducing respiratory drive) and hypoxic ventilatory decline. If hypoxia persists, there is a gradual increase in ventilation which can take several weeks to finally adjust. This acclimatization will result in only a partial correction of the arterial PaO_2.

Table 12.1 The variation in inspired PO_2 with increasing altitude

Altitude		Barometric pressure (kPa)	Inspired gas PO_2 (kPa)
(m)	(ft)		
0	0	101	19.9
1200	4000	87.4	17.0
1800	6000	82.0	15.9
2400	8000	75.2	14.4
3000	10 000	69.7	13.3
6000	20 000	46.5	8.4
9000	30 000	30.1	4.9
12 000	40 000	18.8	2.7

Acclimatization

- There is a respiratory alkalosis with a compensatory metabolic acidosis.
- Erythropoeitin production increases after a few hours to drive increased red cell production which can result in polycythaemia.

- 2,3-Diphosphoglycerate (2, 3-DPG) concentrations increase.
- There is a left shift in the oxygen dissociation curve, increasing oxygen uptake in the lungs at the expense of release to the tissues.

Adaptation

Long-term residents at high altitude have the following developmental changes.
- A blunted ventilatory response to hypoxia and exercise.
- An increased pulmonary diffusion capacity.
- Increased vascularity of cardiac and striated muscle.

Acute medical problems

The problems caused by altitude range from mild symptoms (headaches, fatigue) to life-threatening symptoms (loss of consciousness, cerebral oedema, pulmonary oedema).

Acute hypoxia

Signs/symptoms
- Impaired night vision.
- Reduced mental performance.
- Dyspnoea.
- Loss of consciousness.

Acute mountain sickness (AMS)

Occurs at altitudes >2000 m.

Signs/symptoms
- Headache.
- Dyspnoea.
- Disturbed sleep.
- Fatigue.
- Nausea.
- Poor appetite.

High-altitude pulmonary oedema (HAPE)

- Occurs at altitudes >3000 m in susceptible individuals with an exaggerated increase in pulmonary artery pressure.
- The presentation is that of classical pulmonary oedema (dyspnoea, hypoxia, cough producing pink frothy sputum, and patchy CXR changes).
- Without treatment this carries a high mortality.

High-altitude cerebral oedema (HACE)

Although this is not a respiratory problem, both HACE and HAPE can present in the same patient. Alterations in cerebral blood flow result in cerebral oedema, intracranial thrombosis, and haemorrhage.
- Early signs
  - Irritability.
  - Ataxia.
  - Irrational behaviour.

- Late signs
  - Hallucinations.
  - Drowsiness.
  - Coma.

⚠ Both HAPE and HACE are life-threatening.

Treatment involves the following.

- Supplemental oxygen.
- Reduce altitude quickly (or use a pressurized chamber).
- For HAPE: nifedipine 20 mg bd (10 mg sublingual loading dose).
- For HACE: dexamethasone 4 mg qds (10 mg loading dose).

Acclimatization reduces the likelihood of developing AMS, HACE, and HAPE. This is achieved by a slow controlled ascent. Most of the symptoms of acute mountain sickness will resolve in a few days at the same altitude.

Acetazolamide can be used to accelerate the acclimatization process prior to the onset of symptoms or once mild symptoms of AMS develop. Nifedipine can be used as prophylaxis for HAPE, particularly if an individual has previously been affected. It does not remove the need for a controlled ascent to reduce the risks.

Sleep disturbance

At altitudes >3000 m some individuals demonstrate a periodic breathing pattern during sleep. Given the low oxygen tension already present, this gives rise to profound hypoxaemia and sleep disturbance.

The immunocompromised patient

Introduction

Acute respiratory disease is common in the immunocompromised population who include patients receiving cytotoxic chemotherapy or immunosuppressive therapy for non-malignant conditions (e.g. steroids, cyclophosphamide, azathioprine, methotrexate), recipients of organ transplants, patients with lymphoproliferative or myeloproliferative malignancies, and those with congenital or acquired immunodeficiencies. For a more detailed discussion see OHRM, Chapters 9 and 10.

Common treatment points

- Presentation is usually with dry cough, dyspnoea, fevers, and sweats, often with hypoxia and sometimes chest pain, weight loss, and fatigue.
- Symptoms and signs localizing to the respiratory system can be minimal.
- This discussion will focus on early assessment and treatment of emergencies, as later management should be under the guidance of the patient's main team (e.g. transplant team, HIV consultant, oncologist, etc.) and a respiratory physician.
- 75% of respiratory disease in the immunocompromised is infective and secondary infection with a new organism can occur.
- Bacteraemia is more common.
- Non-infectious causes include pulmonary oedema, pulmonary embolism, diffuse alveolar haemorrhage, ARDS, drug- or radiation-induced pneumonitis, post-transplant lymphoproliferative disease, graft versus host disease in stem cell transplant, and direct involvement of the underlying disease.

① Clinical assessment

History

Features from the history may point to the aetiology and hence management:

Timing of onset of symptoms and its relation to the initial insult
- Acute onset (<24 hours) may indicate bacterial or viral pneumonia, pulmonary oedema (inflammatory or left atrial hypertension), pulmonary haemorrhage, PE, ARDS.
- Subacute onset (days) may indicate fungi (e.g. *Pneumocystis, Aspergillus*), other bacteria (e.g. *Nocardia, Legionella*), viruses (e.g. CMV), idiopathic or drug-induced pneumonitis.
- Chronic onset (weeks) may indicate malignancy, mycobacteria, fungi.
- Radiation pneumonitis typically develops 4–8 weeks after radiotherapy.

Type of immunological defect

- Neutrophil abnormalities (cytotoxics, leukaemia, aplastic anaemia): bacteria, fungi.
- T-cell abnormalities (cytotoxics, post-transplant, HIV, high-dose steroids, lymphoma): fungi, viruses especially CMV, mycobacteria, *Pneumocystis*.
- B-cell or immunoglobulin abnormalities (myeloma, lymphocytic leukaemia, lymphoma): encapsulated bacteria (*Streptococcus pneumoniae, Haemophilus influenzae*).

Duration and severity of the immunological defect

- Mild (e.g. steroids, >6 months after transplantation): there is increased risk of infection with usual community-acquired organisms (*S.pneumoniae, H.influenzae, Staphylococcus aureus*, influenza, RSV), and there is still increased risk of opportunistic infections (viral and bacterial).
- Moderate (e.g. 1–6 months after transplantation, CD4 <200): opportunistic pathogens are common (CMV, *Pneumocystis, Listeria, Nocardia, Aspergillus*, mycobacteria, fungi such as *Aspergillus, Cryptococcus*, and endemic mycoses).
- Severe (e.g. <1 month after transplantation): hospital-acquired organisms from surgery and ITU (*S.aureus*, MRSA, *Klebsiella, Legionella, Pseudomonas*).
- Is the patient taking HAART or prophylaxis against CMV or *Pneumocystis*?

Examination and investigation

- Check SaO_2 and ABGs as hypoxia is often worse than suspected. Monitor pulse, blood pressure, respiratory rate, respiratory effort. Assess fluid status.
- CXR may show consolidation, diffuse infiltrates, or nodularity. Previous radiology may be useful. CT may help if CXR non-diagnostic.
- Haemoptysis may complicate infection, particularly with fungi, or may indicate neoplastic spread.
- Look for extra-pulmonary manifestations of disease (e.g. hepatitis, retinitis, and colitis with CMV).
- Check FBC, U&Es, LFT, amylase, CRP, blood cultures, serology or antigen tests (e.g. CMV, HSV, RSV, urinary *Legionella* antigen), CD4 count if HIV positive.
- Check levels of immunosuppressants if relevant (cyclosporin, tacrolimus).
- Sputum should be sent for fungal staining and culture, *Pneumocystis*, mycobacterial staining and culture and for MC&S.
- Induced sputum for PCP is helpful in HIV.

Management

- Supportive care with fluid balance, oxygen (keep SaO_2 >95%) and ventilatory requirements must be met. Consultation with ITU should occur early if the patient is very unwell or rapidly worsening and likely to require ventilatory support.
- Do not withdraw or adjust immunosuppressants without discussion with the relevant team.
- Investigate and treat pulmonary oedema and pulmonary embolus, as indicated clinically.
- Commence immediate broad-spectrum antibiotic cover for any patient with neutropenia or who is too unwell to await definitive diagnosis. Suggestions are made here, but local hospital policy should be followed:
  - Gram-positive cover (e.g. piperacillin/tazobactam (Tazocin®) 4.5 g IV tds, meropenem 0.5–1 g qds) and Gram-negative cover (e.g. gentamicin 3–5 mg/kg or netilmicin 4–6 mg/kg od).
  - Vancomycin in addition if MRSA suspected.
  - Anti-fungals if no improvement after 2 days (e.g. amphotericin B and itraconazole for *Aspergillus*) or if CT indicates fungal disease likely (irregular nodules, ground-glass opacities and pleural effusions).
- PCP, CMV, HSV and RSV treatment should only be started after diagnosis, but start empirically if patient too unwell to wait.
  - *PCP* CXR may show perihilar shadowing or be relatively normal for degree of hypoxia. Co-trimoxazole 120 mg/kg/day in four divided doses; dilute 480 mg ampoules in 75 ml 5% dextrose and infuse over 60 minutes Change to oral once clinically improving. Prednisolone 20–60 mg od may help in PCP associated with HIV or ventilatory failure.
  - *CMV* At risk patients include seropositive recipients and seronegative recipient with seropositive donors. May be asymptomatic or have fulminant pneumonia with extrathoracic disease. CXR may show diffuse shadows. Treat with ganciclovir 5 mg/kg IV bd for 2–4 weeks.
  - *HSV* Treat with aciclovir.
  - *RSV* Treat with ribavirin.
- Steroids (20–40 mg/day oral, or 10–500 mg IV methylprednisolone) are sometimes used empirically in diffuse alveolar haemorrhage or severe drug- or radiation-induced lung disease, ideally only once infection has been ruled out.
- Early consultation with respiratory and infectious disease physicians will help appropriate timing and use of other investigations (chest CT, bronchoscopy, lung biopsy).

Post lung transplant

ⓘ Common treatment points

This discussion will focus on diagnosis and treatment of emergencies, as later management will be based on consultation with transplant and respiratory teams. For more information see OHRM Chapter 31.

- Patients may have undergone single lung transplant, bilateral sequential lung transplant, or heart–lung transplant, and would usually be discharged about 1 month after surgery.
- Common immunosuppressants used: ciclosporin, sirolimus, tacrolimus, mycophenolate, azathioprine, prednisolone.
- Ciliary function, cough reflex, blood supply, and lymphatic drainage are abnormal in the transplanted lung, predisposing to infection and injury, but oxygenation should be normal by the time of discharge. Donor lung has no bronchial circulation and relies on pulmonary vessels.
- Risk of death and of emergency complications is greatest in year one.
- Survival is 85% at 1 month, 75% at 1 year, 60% at 3 years.
- Discussion with the transplant centre should occur immediately.

Clinical assessment

- Assessment and management are broadly the same as described in the immunosuppression section; early diagnosis is often very difficult. Infection versus rejection is usually diagnosed later on bronchoscopy.
- Include spirometry at the earliest opportunity, as this will inform discussion with the transplant team. FEV_1, FVC, and TLCO rise during first 3 months. Decline is non-specific (it may indicate airway or parenchymal disease) but is helpful to assess severity and response to treatment.
- Measure levels of ciclosporin, sirolimus, or tacrolimus.
- Before prescribing, check for interactions with immunosuppressants.

Complications

Complications within 1 month

Infection

- See notes on immunosuppression.
- Bacterial infection occurs in up to 35%, and is commonly due to Gram-negative organisms (e.g. *Pseudomonas aeruginosa, Enterobacter*).
- Viral pneumonia occurs in 10%.

Pulmonary oedema

- Correct fluid balance if due to volume overload.
- May be due to increased permeability or inflammatory injury.

Acute rejection

- Occurs in 50–75% of patients. Usually within first 3 months, after which other causes of dyspnoea are more likely.
- May be silent in 15–20% of patients, but usually presents with fever, malaise, cough, dyspnoea, hypoxia, and CXR infiltrates (often perihilar and lower lobe shadows with septal lines and pleural fluid).
- Most reliable sign is a fall in FEV_1 >10%.
- Discuss with transplant team. Treatment is usually 3 days of high-dose methylprednisolone after transbronchial biopsies.

Anastamotic stenosis

- Occurs weeks or months after transplant
- Causes wheeze, recurrent infection, reduction in spirometry.
- Diagnosed with CT or bronchoscopy.

Graft versus host disease
Immediate post-operative complications

These, in general, will have been dealt with before discharge but some may very rarely present on-call. Discussion with transplant team is essential before treating. Problems include the following

- Re-implantation injury (usually remits by day 10), early graft dysfunction, hyperacute rejection, anastamotic breakdown, wound infection, haemorrhage, wound dehiscence, phrenic nerve injury, pulmonary artery compression/stenosis.
- Pulmonary emboli: assess and treat in the usual way.
- Pneumothorax: may occur as a surgical complication or due to invasive procedures. Treat as for secondary pneumothorax (📖p. 170 – *pneumothorax algorithm*).
- Pleural effusion: most commonly benign due to smaller size of donor lung. Usually treated conservatively. If symptoms indicate (respiratory compromise, circulatory compromise, or sepsis), perform pleural aspiration with measurement of protein, LDH, glucose levels, and pH using blood gas syringe (unless fluid purulent or contains debris). Send aspirate in blood culture bottles and plain tube for MC&S. If bloodstained, send some in an EDTA blood tube for FBC. Haemothorax is indicated by fluid haematocrit >50% of blood haematocrit. May occur as a complication of surgery or invasive procedures. Ensure adequate circulating volume and insert chest drain. Chylothorax is indicated by milky fluid with high triglycerides (>1.24 mM) and low cholesterol. May occur due to damage of the thoracic duct in surgery. Drain only if causing significant distress. Pus, pH <7.2, low glucose, or high LDH may indicate pleural infection, for which drainage and broad-spectrum antibiotics will be needed.

Complications after 1 month

Infection

- See notes on immunosuppression (📖 Chapter 13).
- Gram-negative organisms are still more common. Therefore, if known or suspected, cover with oral ciprofloxacin or IV third-generation cephalosporin plus an aminoglycoside.
- Opportunistic infection occurs in 35–60% of patients, but may not affect mortality. CMV is the most common.
- Colonization with *Aspergillus* is common, but active infection is rare. May cause anastomotic infection, pneumonia, bronchitis with airway pseudomembrane formation and ulceration, or disseminated disease.
- Risk of viral pneumonia continues undiminished.

Chronic rejection (or 'obliterative bronchiolitis')

- Progressive airway obstruction and bronchiectasis (probably due to repeated injury from microaspiration, chronic rejection, and microorganisms) causing exertional wheeze and dyspnoea.
- Peak incidence in first 2 years, but prevalence increases with time (60–80% affected by 5–10 years).
- May present with recurrent acute bronchitis. Treat with bronchodilators, maintain oxygenation, check ABG if ventilatory insufficiency suspected (e.g. if SaO_2 <93%). Give antibiotics as for acute exacerbation of COPD, but see note above about Gram-negative organisms.

Cryptogenic organizing pneumonia (COP)

- Up to 10% develop COP as part of chronic rejection.
- Presents with fever, cough, hypoxia, and peripheral consolidation.
- Treat with steroids (e.g. prednisolone 40 mg/day) and taper over months.

Post-transplant lymphoproliferative disease

- Peak incidence within first year. Affects 4–10%.
- B-cell proliferation often affects the transplanted lungs (lymphadenopathy, pulmonary infiltrates or pulmonary nodules) and may cause peripheral lymphadenopathy, tonsillar enlargement, or skin nodules. Often associated with EBV infection. Treated with aciclovir and reduced immunosuppression.
- T-cell proliferation may occur later and has poorer prognosis.

Renal impairment due to immunosuppressants
Recurrence

Recurrence of the disease which necessitated the transplant may occur, but rarely causes acute illness.

Chapter 15

Superior vena cava obstruction (SVCO)

① Introduction

Direct invasion of the SVC or compression of the vessel wall by right upper lobe tumours and/or mediastinal lymphadenopathy is the most common mechanism by which this syndrome can arise. Thrombosis within the SVC (which can occur together with direct invasion) is less common.

The cause in >90% is lung cancer (SCLC more commonly than NSCLC; present at diagnosis in 10% SCLC and 1.7% NSCLC) or lymphoma (more frequently NHL). Other rarer causes include mediastinal spread from other primary cancers (e.g. breast), thymoma, and germ cell tumours of the mediastinum. Rarer non-malignant causes include fibrosing mediastinitis.

Presentation

- Dyspnoea.
- Headache.
- Facial plethora.
- Venous distension in the neck and distended veins on the upper chest and arms.
- Upper limb oedema.
- Symptoms from the primary cause may be present to varying degrees.

☼ Evaluation

In the absence of respiratory compromise (e.g. stridor from associated large airway compression) steps to establish a precise tissue diagnosis should be taken prior to starting treatment. High-dose steroids (for which there are no data confirming effectiveness) can cause dramatic shrinkage of mediastinal lymph nodes in lymphoma, making subsequent biopsy technically difficult, along with altering histological appearance of biopsies hampering diagnostic precision. Similar problems exist in establishing a precise diagnosis after radiotherapy.

CXR

May show mediastinal widening and may demonstrate evidence of an underlying lung primary.

CT scanning

All patients with SVCO should have a contrast-enhanced CT scan of chest and upper abdomen as a minimum (ideally include the neck and lower abdomen/pelvis for suspected lymphoma). This will clarify a clinical diagnosis of SVCO along with providing information as to the likely underlying cause and extent of disease.

Tissue diagnosis

CT thorax may show a relatively straightforward site for obtaining histology/ cytology (pleural fluid, supraclavicular lymphadenopathy) but ultimately mediastinal lymph nodes or tumour mass may be the only potential biopsy site. Approach may be possible under CT guidance or with transbronchial needle aspiration at bronchoscopy. However, mediastinoscopy by a thoracic surgeon may be needed (safe in the absence of tracheal obstruction or pericardial effusion).

Establishing a complete diagnosis in lymphoma requires good tissue samples (core biopsy) and FNA cytology is not adequate for this.

Management

In patients presenting with SVCO *de novo*, admission to establish a precise diagnosis is usually warranted before initiating any treatment.

Known diagnosis of lung cancer

Start steroids (dexamethasone 8 mg bd or 4 mg qds) and arrange CT thorax. Refer to respiratory/oncology team looking after the patient for consideration of SVC stenting and/or palliative radiotherapy depending on CT appearances. Prompt outpatient management is often adequate.

Palliative radiotherapy ± chemotherapy is often first-line approach to management of SVCO caused by lung cancer. In SCLC, prompt chemotherapy without radiotherapy may be adequate.

Intraluminal stenting can be used as a primary treatment in NSCLC and may provide more rapid relief of symptoms than radiotherapy.[1] In SCLC chemotherapy is usually the first-line treatment. Stenting is particularly important in recurrent SVCO where further oncological treatment may not be possible or successful.

Known diagnosis of lymphoma

Discuss with haematology/oncology team looking after patient in first instance before commencing steroid treatment. Systemic chemotherapy (with or without radiotherapy) is the treatment of choice. The role of intraluminal stenting in lymphoma is more controversial.

---

1 Rowell NP, Gleeson FV (2001). Steroids, radiotherapy, chemotherapy and stents for superior vena caval obstruction in carcinoma of the bronchus. *Cochrane Database Syst Rev*, **4**, CD001316.

End-stage pulmonary disease

⊘ End-stage pulmonary disease

The WHO defines palliative care as the active total care of patients whose disease is not responsive to curative treatment. The goal of palliative care is achievement of best quality of life for patients and their families. It includes control of pain and other physical symptoms as well as care of psychological, social and spiritual problems.

Within respiratory medicine, patients with lung malignancy are the group most often considered for palliative support, but many other patients with progressive respiratory disease (e.g. COPD, diffuse interstitial lung disease, bronchiectasis, and CF) will also benefit. In addition to specific medical therapies for symptoms, a multidisciplinary approach to offer practical support and anxiety management is indicated.

Symptoms for palliation

Pain

- Assess fully as to cause of pain.
- Treat initially with simple oral analgesia, incrementing treatment according to the WHO three analgesic stepladder (non-opioid analgesia, then weak opioids, then strong opioids) until adequate pain control.
- Prescribe adequate doses of analgesia and titrate dose accordingly.
- Ensure patient has analgesia for breakthrough pain.
- Think about alternative routes if unable to take oral medication.
- Treat side effects such as constipation and nausea effectively.
- Think about adjuvant analgesics for specific types of pain (Table 16.1).
- Consider referral to pain clinic for further interventions such as nerve blocks and transcutaneous electrical nerve stimulation (TENS).

Dyspnoea

- Breathlessness is a common symptom and is exacerbated by pain and anxiety.
- Opioids (e.g. oral morphine sulphate 2.5–5 mg) are very effective at relieving the sensation of dyspnoea without affecting respiratory function.
- If breathlessness seems disproportionate to level of underlying disease, or abruptly deteriorates, consider other possible causes (see box).
- Short burst oxygen is often beneficial.

Table 16.1 Common adjuvant analgesics for cancer pain

Drug	Indication
Non-steroidal anti-inflammatory drugs	Bone pain
	Soft tissue infiltration
	Hepatomegaly
Corticosteriods	Raised intracranial pressure
	Soft tissue infiltration
	Nerve compression
	Hepatomegaly
Antidepressants (e.g. amitryptyline)	Nerve compression
Anticonvulsants (e.g. gabapentin)	Paraneoplastic neuropathies
Bisphosphanates	Bone pain

Causes of breathlessness in lung cancer and their treatment

Lung tumour	Radiotherapy or chemotherapy
Bronchospasm	Bronchodilators
Infection	Antibiotics
Pleural effusion	Pleural drain and pleurodesis
Anaemia	Blood transfusion
Pulmonary emboli	Anticoagulation
Lymphangitis	Corticosteroids
Upper airway obstruction	Stent or brachytherapy
SVCO	SVC stent
Pericardial effusion	Pericardial drain

Other symptoms

Cough

- Very common and can be debilitating.
- Look for reversible causes such as infection or bronchospasm and treat accordingly.
- If no reversible cause found try simple or codeine linctus. If cough persists, oral codeine or opiates act as cough suppressants and may be of benefit.
- Nebulized local anaesthetic can help (5 ml 2% lidocaine). There is a risk of aspiration 1 hour after treatment due to pharyngeal numbness so avoid fluids during this period.
- Diazepam can also be used as a central cough depressant especially if associated anxiety.

Anxiety

- Causes dyspnoea which worsens anxiety (leading to vicious circle).
- Benzodiazepines (e.g. lorazepam 2–4 mg sublingually) often useful.
- Midazolam best for acute panic; given IV initially 2–2.5 mg then incremental doses of 1 mg.
- Antidepressants (e.g. amitriptyline and SSRIs) are useful anxiolytics.
- Complementary therapies may be helpful (e.g. aromatherapy, hypnosis, massage, relaxation techniques).

Haemoptysis (□ Chapter 6)

- Can be extremely frightening and occasionally catastrophic.
- Palliative radiotherapy may be useful.
- Oral anti-fibrinolytics such as tranexamic acid may help.
- Interventional bronchoscopy with diathermy is becoming more commonly available.

Superior vena cava obstruction (□ Chapter 15)

- Presents with facial swelling.
- Diagnosis confirmed using thoracic CT with contrast.
- Start on high-dose dexamethasone (e.g. 8 mg bd).
- Refer to interventional radiologist for insertion of SVC stent.

Poor appetite

- Common symptom due to anorexia or mouth problems, nausea, hypercalcaemia, drugs, or depression.
- May be improved in the short term by course of oral steroids, such as prednisolone 10 mg od for 4 weeks.
- Consider nutritional supplements.

Post thoracic surgery

① Post thoracic surgery

Successful post-operative management of the thoracic surgical patient requires careful assessment. Potential complications should be recognized and managed early, as this will reduce post-operative morbidity and mortality.

Post-operative complications

- In current clinical practice 30 day postoperative mortality following elective lobectomy is approximately 2–3% and minor morbidity is 40–50%.
- For pneumonectomy, mortality is 6–8% and minor morbidity is 35–75%.
- Extended pulmonary resection involving chest wall and pericardium is associated with increased mortality of up to 20%.
- Main causes of mortality and morbidity are from respiratory and cardiac causes.
- Patients should be assessed and investigations done accordingly (see below).
- Need early communication with surgical team.

Respiratory complications

Respiratory problems are the most commonest cause of postoperative morbidity and mortality. Respiratory failure occurs in up to 2% of patients. Main causes include the following.

Pneumonia

- Aspiration and impaired host defences cause reduced mucociliary clearance and impaired cough reflex, resulting in atelectasis.
- Can happen within 48 hours of operation or later.
- Presents with fever, dyspnoea, and chest pain. CXR shows consolidation.
- Management includes antibiotics, analgesia, and chest physiotherapy.
- In severe cases, respiratory support may be required.

Lobar gangrene

- This occurs when there is torsion of the remaining lobe resulting in vascular and bronchial obstruction causing pulmonary infarction and lobar gangrene.
- Usually presents within 48 hours of operation but can happen up to 7 days afterwards.
- Presents with fever and haemoptysis. Serial CXRs show an increase in parenchymal opacification.
- If torsion is suspected, need to take back to theatre early for exploration to prevent permanent damage.
- If ischaemic injury is severe lobectomy will be required.

Pulmonary embolism

- Commonly occurs 10–14 days after operation.
- High index of suspicion is required to make diagnosis.
- Presents classically with dyspnoea and pleuritic chest pain.
- Can be difficult to differentiate clinically from pneumonia.
- Confirm diagnosis with CTPA.
- Treat with anticoagulation.

Bronchopleural fistula

- Occurs in approximately 3% of patients.
- May indicate recurrence of tumour.
- Usually associated with an infected pleural space.
- Results in persistent sepsis, failure of re-expansion of the remaining lung, and contamination of the contralateral lung.
- Presents with fever and a productive cough, often postural.
- CXR may show an air fluid level.
- Manage with respiratory support and IV antibiotics.
- Need early liaison with respiratory and surgical team to consider bronchoscopy and drainage of space.
- If bronchoscopy confirms a fistula, further surgery is likely to be necessary.

Cardiac complications

These usually occur perioperatively. They include the following.
- Cardiac failure.
- Myocardial infarction.
- Cardiac dysarrhythmias.

Investigations

- ABGs.
- CXR: may show infiltrates with pneumonia and lobar gangrene or air/fluid level with development of a bronchopleural fistula.
- ECG: useful in diagnosis of an acute myocardial infarction and pulmonary embolism, which may show features of right heart strain.
- CT thorax: allows the lungs to be assessed in more detail and looks for pulmonary emboli.
- Pleural aspiration: for suspected bronchopleural fistula, but discuss with thoracic surgeon before doing this.
- Bronchoscopy: useful to look at bronchial stump and whether it is intact.
- CTPA: if pulmonary emboli expected.

Part 3

Acute respiratory conditions

Anaphylaxis

☠ Anaphylaxis

Anaphylactic reactions (type I hypersensitivity reaction) are the consequence of the cascade caused by an IgE-mediated response to a specific antigen. Prior exposure to the antigen sensitizes the individual, so that subsequent exposure results in prostaglandin, leukotriene, and platelet activating factor generation and thereby histamine release. This results in vasodilatation, bronchial mucosal oedema, and bronchoconstriction.

A number of antigens can be responsible for anaphylaxis. Common causes are foodstuffs (peanuts, eggs), latex, bee/wasp stings, blood products and drugs (vaccinations, aspirin, penicillin).

Features
- Erythema/urticaria.
- Facial/oropharyngeal mucosal oedema.
- Stridor.
- Wheeze.
- Tachypnoea.
- Warm peripheries/peripheral vasodilatation.
- Hypotension.
- Tachycardia.

▶▶ Treatment
- ABC.
- High-flow oxygen.
- Secure airway if there are signs of airway compromise. Cricothyroidotomy may be required if airway swelling makes intubation impossible.
- Adrenaline IM 0.5 mg (0.5 ml of 1:1000), repeated after 5 minutes if hypotension persists.
- Chlorphenamine 10–20 mg IV.
- Hydrocortisone 100–300 mg IV.
- IV fluid resuscitation if hypotensive.
- Nebulized bronchodilators (salbutamol 2.5–5 mg) or IV adrenaline (5 ml of 1:10 000).

⚠ IV adrenaline should be avoided except where there is significant circulatory compromise and hence doubt about absorption from an intramuscular site. IV adrenaline is administered as **5 ml of 1:10 000 strength** (0.5 mg) at a rate of **1 ml/minute, stopping when there is a response.**

- Observe for 12 hours as there can be a deterioration some hours after the initial event.
- Continue oral chlorphenamine 4 mg qds for 24–48 hours.
- Continue steroids (oral prednisolone 30–40 mg od) for 24–48 hours.
- Pre-filled adrenaline syringe for self-administration, together with appropriate education and instruction on using this device (EpiPen®).

Specialist centres can perform specific allergen testing and occasionally allergen immunotherapy is used to desensitize the patient.

C1-esterase inhibitor deficiency (hereditary angio-oedema)

- Autosomal dominant condition.
- Ask about similar crises in other family members.
- Can be mistaken for anaphylaxis.
- Symptoms and signs primarily caused by oedema, including gastrointestinal oedema.
- Check C1-esterase inhibitor and complement levels.

Treatment

- Similar to anaphylaxis.
- Administer C1-esterase inhibitor plasma concentrate 1000–1500 units or fresh frozen plasma.
- May not respond to antihistamines.

Tranexamic acid or danazol are used for long-term prophylaxis.

Acute respiratory distress syndrome (ARDS)

☼ ARDS

Acute respiratory distress syndrome occurs when the lung suffers an insult which results in non-cardiogenic pulmonary oedema and hypoxaemia refractory to oxygen therapy. It was initially termed adult respiratory distress syndrome, but it can occur in infants. The terms acute lung injury (ALI) or shock lung have been used to describe the same process. ALI was defined in the 1994 American-European Consensus conference criteria as a less severe form of ARDS.

The full definition of ARDS/ALI is diffuse pulmonary infiltrates, refractory hypoxaemia, decreased lung compliance, and respiratory distress. The definition includes measurement of pulmonary artery pressure to distinguish ARDS/ALI from cardiac causes of lungs infiltrates and refractory hypoxaemia.

Criteria required to diagnose ARDS/ALI

- Acute onset.
- Bilateral infiltrates on CXR.
- Pulmonary capillary wedge pressure <18 mmHg or no evidence of left atrial hypertension. Echocardiography is helpful to establish LV function.
- Refractory hypoxaemia
  - ALI ratio $PaO_2:FiO_2$ <300 mmHg (40 kPa).
  - ARDS ratio $PaO_2:FiO_2$ <200 mmHg (27 kPa).

Pathophysiology

The initial insult results in increased vascular permeability secondary to microcirculatory changes and production of inflammatory mediators. This results in pulmonary interstitial oedema, damage to the pulmonary epithelium, and reduction in surfactant production. Initially vascular compression from pulmonary interstitial oedema, and then increased autonomic nervous activity, results in pulmonary hypertension. Ventilation – perfusion mismatching occurs contributing to refractory hypoxaemia.

An exudate forms within the alveoli. This contains an abundance of clotting factors, platelets, fibrin, and fibrinogen. This inactivates surfactant and promotes hyaline membrane formation. Fibroblastic proliferation results in lung fibrosis.

Symptoms and signs

Any relating to the cause for ARDS plus:

- Tachypnoea.
- Hypoxia.
- Tachycardia.
- Agitation, lethargy.
- Coarse inspiratory crackles.
- CXR shows pulmonary infiltrates in an alveolar pattern. This can be patchy or unilateral initially. There may also be air bronchograms. Later stages show the more typical 'white-out'.

Table 19.1 Causes of ARDS/ALI

Direct	Indirect
Pneumonia	Sepsis
Smoke/toxic inhalation	Massive trauma
Gastric aspiration	Transfusion of blood products
Near drowning	Burns
Lung contusion	Acute pancreatitis
Amniotic fluid embolus	Cardiopulmonary bypass
Fat emboli	Eclampsia
	DIC
	DKA
	Drugs, e.g. opiates, aspirin
	Head injury/raised ICP

Management

Treat the underlying cause. Treatment for ARDS is supportive.

- ABG assessment of hypoxaemia and PCO_2 (low initially but hypercapnia develops as respiratory failure worsens).
- CPAP (5–10 cmH$_2$O) with 100% O_2 may help hypoxaemia but is often only a temporary solution.
- Intubation and ventilation (low volume 6 ml/kg, permissive hypercapnia) is indicated if there is any of the following:
  - acidosis.
  - exhaustion.
  - hypoxaemia.
  - reduced conscious level.
- Cautious IV fluid support as excessive administration will worsen the pulmonary oedema.
- Culture any potential infective source (sputum/BAL, urine, blood). Broad-spectrum antibiotics are frequently given. Inflammatory markers and WCC are likely to be raised in ARDS even in the absence of infection.
- CVP, cardiac output, and mixed venous oxygen saturation monitoring.
- Inotropic support and renal replacement therapy are frequently required as ARDS commonly results in multi-organ failure.
- Enteral feeding via a NG tube is recommended.
- Ventilating the patient in the prone position for several hours can improve oxygenation. This improves perfusion to aerated areas of the lung. Inverse ratio ventilation (inspiration > expiration) can also be used.

A number of other treatments have been trialled in ARDS but there is limited evidence of a survival benefit.
- Surfactant replacement.
- Corticosteroids.
- Inhaled nitric oxide.
- Nebulized epoprostenol.
- Extra-corporeal membrane oxygenation.
- High frequency jet ventilation.
- Liquid ventilation with perfluorocarbons.

Prognosis

This is dependent upon the initial insult causing ARDS. Mortality is about 60%. Increasing age and multiple organ failure are poor prognostic markers. Survivors may have a degree of pulmonary fibrosis and a restrictive pattern on pulmonary function testing.

Asthma

Definition

'Asthma is a chronic inflammatory disorder of the airways in which many cells and cellular components play a role. The chronic inflammation causes an associated increase in airway hyper-responsiveness that leads to recurrent episodes of wheezing, breathlessness, chest tightness and coughing, particularly at night or in the early morning. These episodes are usually associated with widespread but variable airflow obstruction that is often reversible either spontaneously or with treatment.' (GINA Workshop 2005: www.ginaasthma.org,uk)

The prevalence of asthma is increasing, more so in children than adults, with the WHO estimating that there are currently 100–150 million people worldwide with asthma, with approximately 180 000 deaths per year. Highest levels of asthma are seen in the developed countries. It is the most common chronic respiratory condition in the UK with a prevalence of 10–15%.

In the UK there are peaks of asthma deaths, in the summer in younger patients and in the winter in older patients.

☠ Symptoms and signs

Symptoms
- Wheeze.
- SOB.
- Chest tightness.
- Cough.

These symptoms tend to be:
- Variable.
- Intermittent.
- Worse at night and/or early morning.
- Triggered. Common triggers include:
  - Allergens.
  - Respiratory infections.
  - Irritants.
  - Weather.
  - Exercise.
  - Medication.
  - Emotional stress.

Other features
- Family (or personal) history of asthma or atopy.
- Worsening symptoms with medication, e.g. aspirin or beta-blockers.
- Be aware of occupational asthma. Ask if symptoms are better at weekends or holidays.

Signs
- None.
- Wheeze: diffuse, polyphonic, expiratory, bilateral.
- May have reduced peak flow/FEV_1 (normal between exacerbations).

Diagnosis

This is a clinical diagnosis based on a combination of symptoms and confirmatory objective measures.

Objective measurements

≥15% diurnal variation on >3 days in a week for 2 weeks on PEF diary

OR

↑ ≥15% FEV_1 (or 200 ml) performed 20 minutes after short-acting β_2 agonist (either salbutamol MDI 200 mcg via spacer or 2.5 mg via nebulizer)

OR

↑ ≥15% FEV_1 (or 200 ml) after 14 day steroid trial (prednisolone 30 mg/day).

OR

↓ ≥15% FEV_1 after 6 minutes exercise.

- Can use methacholine or histamine challenge in difficult cases.

Differential diagnosis
- COPD.
- Cardiac disease.
- Tumour:
  - lung
  - tracheal
  - laryngeal.
- Foreign body.
- Bronchiectasis.
- Interstitial lung disease.
- PE.
- Aspiration.
- Vocal cord dysfunction.
- Hyperventilation.

✸ Management of acute asthma

History
- There is often a history of symptoms suggesting worsening asthma in the preceding few days.
  - Increasing use of β_2 agonist, including overnight.
  - Nocturnal cough.
  - Early morning chest tightness.
- Obtain information on background asthma control (before this attack).
  - Frequency of daily use of short-acting β_2 agonist.
  - Number of prior admissions to hospital over past year.
  - Prior admissions to ITU.
  - Best PEF if known (within last 2 years).
- Look for trigger factors.
  - Associated infection.
  - Known allergen.
  - Change in asthma medication (or run out), or introduction of new medication (e.g. NSAIDs or beta-blockers).

Examination
- Observations:
  - SaO_2.
  - Respiratory rate.
  - Heart rate.
  - Blood pressure.
  - Temperature.
- PEF measurement: pre-nebulizer.
- Auscultation of chest.

Investigations
- FBC.
- Theophylline level, if usually taken.
- CXR (to exclude pneumothorax and to look for infection).
- ABG if SaO_2 <92%.

Grading of severity of the acute exacerbation and subsequent management is guided by the PEF recording and examination of the patient for pulse, BP, RR, ability to complete sentences, and air entry.
- Mild: PEF ≥75% predicted.
- Moderate: PEF 50–75% predicted.
- Severe: PEF 33–50% predicted.
- ▶▶ Life-threatening: PEF <33% predicted.

If the patient is seen in the community (or A&E), admit if PEF <50% or there are concerns regarding ability to respond to symptoms, social concerns, exacerbation occurring late in the day, or prior history of brittle asthma.

Those patients who are at increased risk of death from asthma include:
- Those with severe asthma.
- Known brittle asthma or previous near fatal asthma.
- Those with severe asthma and adverse behavioural or psychosocial features, including:
  - Non-compliance, previous self-discharge.
  - Psychiatric illness.
  - Social isolation.
  - Alcohol or drug abuse.
  - Learning difficulties.
  - Obesity.

All patients with asthma should have (if required):
- High-flow oxygen.
- Nebulized bronchodilators driven by oxygen, or bronchodilators given via MDI and spacer.

Management algorithms[1]

Mild exacerbation
- PEF 75% predicted.
- Give usual bronchodilator
  - In mild-moderate exacerbations β_2 agonist via MDI and spacer device is as effective as a nebulizer.
- Check at 15–30 minutes:
  - PEF ≥75% and clinically stable: no further treatment → observe for 2 hours and discharge if stable (see discharge planning below).
  - PEF ≤75% but clinically stable → treat as moderate exacerbation.

Algorithms for moderate exacerbation, acute severe asthma, and life-threatening asthma are shown in Figs. 20.1, 20.2, and 20.3, respectively.

---

1 Algorithms from the BTS Asthma Guidelines (www.brit-thoracic.org.uk)

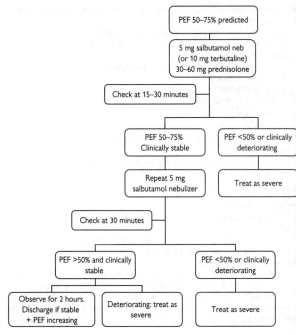

Fig. 20.1 Moderate exacerbation.

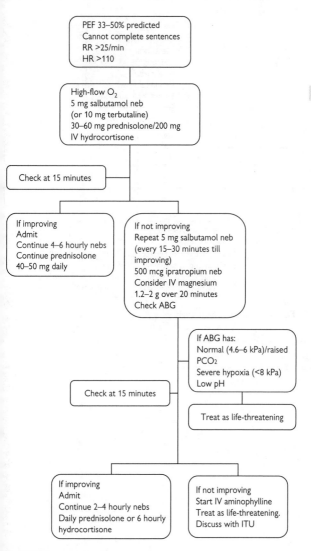

Fig. 20.2 Acute severe asthma.

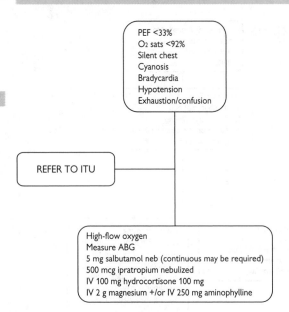

Fig. 20.3 Life-threatening asthma.

Asthma in pregnancy

- Acute asthma should be treated as per the non-pregnant patient: asthma medications are regarded as safe in pregnancy and should be continued or initiated without hesitation.
- Risk to mother and fetus are much greater from uncontrolled asthma than from its treatment.
- Maintain oxygen saturations >95% to prevent fetal hypoxia.
- Obstetric advice should be sought: continuous fetal monitoring is recommended in severe asthma.
- 📖 Chapter 4.

Discharge planning

- Patients should be on home medication for 24 hours prior to discharge.
- PEF >75% predicted and <25% variability.

On discharge, all patients should have:
- Prednisolone 40 mg for at least 5 days.
- Oral antibiotics if confirmed evidence of infection.
- Supply of all inhalers and technique checked.
- PEF meter.
- Written self-management plan.
- Advised to see GP or asthma nurse within the next few days.
- Letter to GP re admission.
- Those with severe asthma should be referred for follow-up in the chest clinic. Repeat attendees to A&E should also be considered for referral to optimize their asthma management.

Chronic obstructive pulmonary disease (COPD)

Chronic obstructive pulmonary disease (COPD) is increasing in frequency worldwide, particularly in developed countries, and has a major impact both in terms of mortality and morbidity. In 2004, respiratory disease accounted for 20% of all deaths in the UK, with COPD accounting for more than a fifth of these. Cases of COPD account for up to 12% of acute medical admissions and use more than 1 million bed days a year in the NHS in England. Approximately 95% of cases of COPD are smoking related, with the remainder being secondary to occupational and environmental exposure.

Diagnosis

The diagnosis of COPD is based on symptoms and signs, supported by spirometry. It should be considered in those over 35 years of age with a history of smoking and one or more of the following symptoms.
- Shortness of breath on exertion.
- Chronic cough.
- Regular sputum production.
- Frequent winter 'bronchitis'.
- Wheeze.

Additional symptoms to enquire about include weight loss, ankle swelling, functional limitation and occupational exposure.

Symptoms of diurnal variability, nocturnal predilection for symptoms, young age (<35 years), and eczema and rhinitis should raise the differential diagnosis of asthma.

Spirometry

Spirometry should be performed for diagnosis of COPD.
- Obstructive picture with reduced FEV_1 (<80% predicted) and FEV_1/FVC ratio <70%.
- Pulmonary function tests may also show raised total lung capacity and residual volume due to air trapping, and reduced gas transfer due to emphysema.

:⊕: Acute exacerbations of COPD

An exacerbation is defined as an acute and sustained worsening of symptoms causing a patient to seek medical advice. It is a clinical diagnosis. Common presentations are:
- Deterioration of pre-existing symptoms of shortness of breath.
- Cough.
- Increased sputum production or change in sputum colour.

Causes

Usually infective, either viral or bacterial (typically *Haemophilus influenzae*, *Streptococcus pneumoniae*, and *Moraxella catarrhalis*).

Other differential diagnoses to consider in a patient with COPD presenting with increased shortness of breath are pneumothorax, pulmonary emboli, cardiac dysfunction, lobar or segmental collapse due to sputum retention or tumour.

Assessment of severity

A brief history should be taken to gain an idea of premorbid functional abilities, previous admissions to hospital or intensive care, level of usual treatment (home nebulizers and/or oxygen), and comorbidities.

Respiratory rate >25 and use of accessory muscles indicate respiratory distress. In addition, all patients should have their BP, heart rate, respiratory rate, temperature, and oxygen saturations (ideally on air) recorded.

After initial assessment a decision should be made as to where the patient is best managed.

Table 21.1 Decision to treat at home or in hospital

Factor	Treat at home	Treat in hospital
SOB	Mild	Severe
Speed of onset	Gradual	Rapid
SaO_2 <90%	No	Yes
Acute confusion	Absent	Present
Conscious level	Normal	Impaired
Peripheral oedema	Absent	Present
Social situation	Good	Living alone, not coping
Premorbid level	Good	Poor
Significant comorbidity	No	Yes
CXR changes	No	Yes
Arterial pH	>7.35	<7.35

Investigations

- FBC (anaemia, infection).
- U&Es (dehydration, renal failure, watch K^+).
- Theophylline level if on oral medication.
- Blood cultures if pyrexial.
- Pulse oximetry.
- CXR.
- ABG (to assess pH and to guide oxygen therapy; see below).
- ECG.

Management

24–28% controlled oxygen should be commenced immediately if hypoxic while awaiting ABG.

❶ The aim of oxygen therapy is to maintain SaO_2 between 85% and 90%, a balance between avoiding hypoxia and subsequent anaerobic metabolism and hypercapnia precipitated by too much oxygen. An assessment needs to be made as to whether controlled O_2 is required (📖 Chapter 44).

It is not uncommon to find significant hypercapnia in a patient brought in by ambulance where uncontrolled oxygen has been given; treatment with appropriate controlled oxygen therapy often corrects this.

Non-invasive ventilation (NIV) should be started in those patients with an acute exacerbation of COPD who fail to respond to initial maximal medical therapy and appropriate controlled oxygen therapy with:
- pH <7.35.
- PCO_2 >6.

In most cases, NIV should be commenced at an IPAP of 10–12 mmH_2O, and an EPAP of 4–5 mmH_2O. Oxygen can be entrained to maintain SaO_2 between 85% and 90% and nebulizer treatment should be continued.

Before starting NIV a clear decision should be documented as to whether this is the ceiling of treatment or whether the patient should have invasive ventilation in the event of failure of NIV. NIV is not usually indicated in those with end-stage disease and poor performance status.

There is no indication for the use of doxapram where NIV is readily available.

Nebulized bronchodilators should be administered on arrival (driven on air if there are concerns regarding type 2 respiratory failure).
- 5 mg salbutamol (or 10 mg terbutaline) plus 500 mcg ipratropium bromide.

Steroids (oral prednisolone 30 mg/day or IV hydrocortisone 100 mg 6 hourly if too unwell to have oral medication) should be started in all patients presenting with an exacerbation and should be continued for 7–14 days.

IV aminophylline should be considered in those not responding to nebulizer treatment. Those not on oral theophyllines prior to admission should receive a loading dose followed by a maintenance infusion.
- Loading dose: 5 mcg/kg given in 250 ml 5% dextrose or 0.9% saline over 0.5–1 hour.
- Maintenance dose of 0.5 mg/kg/hour (diluted with 5% dextrose or 0.9% saline).

Patients on IV aminophylline should be placed on a cardiac monitor and theophylline levels should be measured within 24 hours of starting, and then on a daily basis, to guide treatment and prevent toxicity.

Treat cause of exacerbation
- Antibiotics (e.g. amoxicillin) should be started in patients with one or more of the following:
  - Purulent sputum.
  - Pyrexia.
  - CXR changes.
  - Raised white cell count/CRP.
- Exclude pneumothorax: if present treat as secondary pneumothorax (📖 p. 170 – *pneumothorax algorithm*).
- Consider PE (📖 p. 184 – *submassive PE algorithm*).

Early discharge schemes

Many hospitals now have an early discharge COPD team with strict entry criteria for those patients who are appropriate for such a management plan. The aim is to minimize hospital stay and prevent future admissions where possible. Usual criteria for acceptance onto the scheme are:

- No social problems (i.e. can manage at home).
- No consolidation on CXR.
- No severe blood gas abnormalities (e.g. type 2 respiratory failure that may require NIV).
- No other acute comorbidities requiring medical input.

Discharge planning

Consider discharge once the patient is approaching their usual premorbid level of functioning. Inflammatory markers should be normalizing if elevated on admission.

- Patients should be discharged with a short course of oral steroids to complete (usually 7–14 days in total). In some patients a reducing course may be used if they have had several previous recent courses or are on a usual maintenance dose of steroid.
- Inhaler technique should be checked prior to discharge.
- Arrange short-burst oxygen for those who remain symptomatic and hypoxic with a 6 week review for assessment for long-term oxygen therapy (PO_2 <7.3 when stable).
- Smoking cessation advice.
- Social input as required.
- If CXR abnormal on admission, follow up at 6 weeks to ensure changes resolved.
- Consider referral for pulmonary rehabilitation/commence inpatient pulmonary rehabilitation if available.
- Refer to COPD community teams to increase support and try and prevent future admissions.

References

BTS Guidelines on COPD (www.brit-thoracic.org.uk)

Hyperventilation syndrome

ⓘ **Hyperventilation syndrome**

Syndrome characterized by a variety of somatic symptoms induced by inappropriate hyperventilation and reproduced in whole or part by voluntary hyperventilation.

Rapid shallow breathing leads to hypocapnia and respiratory alkalosis which in turn leads to physical symptoms. There is usually inadequate expiration causing symptoms of chest tightness. These symptoms in turn lead to an increase in anxiety and the development of a 'vicious circle'.

❶ Should be distinguished from tachypnoea (an increase in respiratory frequency) and hyperpnoea (an increase in minute ventilation).

Presentation
- Intermittent episodes of breathlessness usually unrelated to exercise but sometimes worsened by exercise.
- Associated symptoms of lightheadedness or dizziness; occasionally loss of consciousness.
- Paraesthesia in finger tips and peri-orally.
- Tetany/carpopedal spasm.
- Often associated with a recent stressful situation such as a bereavement or mild illness.

Differential diagnosis
- Mild interstitial lung disease with normal CXR.
- Mild asthma with normal PFTs.
- Pulmonary hypertension.
- Thromboembolic disease.
- Hyperthyroidism.

Investigations
Need to exclude organic pathology.
- U&Es and LFTs to exclude metabolic cause.
- TFTs to exclude hyperthyroidism.
- ECG and occasionally echocardiography to exclude cardiac cause.
- CXR and PFTs to exclude respiratory cause.
- Exercise oximetry: either walk the patient along the flat or ask them to step up and down a stair while monitoring SaO_2. Development of dyspnoea with a lack of desaturation excludes a respiratory condition.
- A normal SaO_2 at rest and on exercise to the point of breathlessness can be a good confirmatory test and exclude organic disease.
- ABGs: low $PaCO_2$, alkalosis and a normal A–a gradient (📖 Chapter 53 for A–a gradient calculation).

Management

- Discuss with respiratory team. HRCT may be performed to exclude subtle ILD and liaison with specialist respiratory physiotherapist may be considered for exercises to 'reset' breathing pattern.
- If diagnosis is suspected, discuss with patient sensitively and try to identify provoking factors. Reiterate the normal investigations to reassure them.
- A short period of an anxiolytic (e.g. diazepam 2–5 mg) may be helpful to demonstrate that symptoms can be controlled.
- Management of psychological problems may be helpful and referral to a psychologist is sometimes required.
- Prognosis is usually good but symptoms can relapse.

⚠ If symptoms do not settle reconsider organic pathology.

Imported infectious respiratory disease

☼ Avian influenza

There are few avian influenza viruses that have crossed the species barrier to infect humans, all known cases of which have resulted from contact with infected birds. Infected birds shed influenza virus in saliva, nasal secretions, and faeces.

Subtypes of influenza exist due to changes in two surface proteins on the virus.
● Haemagglutinin (16 known subtypes).
● Neuraminidase (9 known subtypes).

H5N1 is a highly pathogenic strain of avian influenza, and has caused the highest number of human cases and deaths of those strains that have crossed the species barrier. Currently, person to person spread is very limited, but this may change with alterations in the virus itself. Transmission in humans would be droplet or airborne spread. There is now evidence that some of the later clinically documented cases of SARS may well have been avian influenza with the H5N1 strain.

February and March are peak influenza season in east Asia; therefore there will be increased numbers of normal human influenza cases around these times.

Total laboratory confirmed cases (at time of print) stand at 228 with 130 deaths across 10 countries.

▶ Currently the mortality of H5N1 avian influenza stands at >50%.

There is no vaccine currently available for H5N1 avian influenza though work is ongoing.

Natural history
Recently reported cases have presented within 2–6 days of symptom onset, with death occurring at 4–10 days.

Differential diagnosis
● Other acute respiratory illness (particularly atypical infections such as *Legionella*).
● SARS.

Laboratory investigations
● Immunofluorescence (IFA) test for influenza A.
● Nasopharyngeal aspirate or throat swab for A/H5 identification via PCR or viral culture.

Case definition

Sudden onset severe (requiring hospitalization) unexplained respiratory illness (or death from respiratory illness) with fever and cough.

AND

Travel in the previous 7 days to a country with H5N1 in the poultry or animal population.

AND

Contact history: at least one of the following in the country above.
- Within 1 m of live/dead fowl or swine or wild birds.
- Exposure to a setting where fowl/swine have been confined in the previous 6 weeks.
- Close contact with a confirmed human case.
- Close contact with a person with an unexplained respiratory illness that led to their death.

Management of suspected case of avian influenza

- Isolate the patient.
  - Given the human to human transmission of droplet or airborne spread this is vital.
  - Ideally negative-pressure room.
- Use high-efficiency masks (FFP3 standard) as well as gown, gloves, and goggles.
- Thorough history, particularly travel and contact history.
- Minimize contact with designated healthcare workers and minimal visitors.
- Seek specialist help: on-call microbiologist and infectious disease consultants.
- Clinical work-up
  - CXR.
  - FBC, U&E, LFT, CRP.
  - Pulse oximetry: ABG in those with SaO_2 <92%.
  - ECG in those with comorbidity.
  - Blood and sputum cultures.
  - *Legionella* and pneumococcal antigen as well as atypical pneumonia serology.
- Send respiratory (NPA or combined nose and throat swab) and blood samples for influenza A and B.
- Instigate supportive care with oxygen, IV fluids, ± broad-spectrum IV antibiotics (as per community-acquired pneumonia guidelines) until diagnosis confirmed.
  - Avoid nebulizers and high-flow oxygen masks where possible as these may increase the risk of airborne spread.
  - Treat as severe pneumonia (using CURB 65 score for guidance).
  - NIV may be helpful in those with COPD or as a precursor to invasive ventilation. Ensure appropriate infection control procedures are in place.

- Start antiviral treatment in those fulfilling case definition criteria. Consider one of the following.
  - Oseltamivir 75 mg bd for 5 days.
  - Zanamavir 10 mg bd for 5 days.
  - No case currently for ribavirin or corticosteroids.
  - H5N1 in Asia has been shown to be resistant to amantadine and rimantidine.
- Consider nutritional support in those with severe illness.
- Refer to ITU those with:
  - Persisting hypoxia (PaO_2 <8) despite maximal oxygen.
  - Worsening hypercapnia.
  - Severe acidosis (pH <7.26).
  - Septic shock.
- Report to CCDC and contact trace.

All healthcare workers in contact with suspected cases should monitor their temperature twice daily. Fever (>38°C) should be reported and prophylaxis instigated if appropriate (oseltamivir 75 mg o.d. for 7 days).

If severity of clinical condition does not warrant hospitalization then they should be treated at home, with isolation precautions, and follow-up by health protection team within 48 hours to confirm recovery. Hospitalize if condition deteriorates.

Further information

www.hpa.org.uk
www.who.int/csr/disease/avian_influenza

☼ Severe acute respiratory syndrome (SARS)

The first case of SARS occurred in the Guandong province of China in November 2002. However, the disease was first recognized as a global threat in March 2003. The last known human transmission occurred in July 2003, by which time 8098 cases had been reported with 774 deaths across 26 countries. Currently (at time of print) we are in an inter-epidemic period.

SARS is caused by a coronavirus, an animal virus that has crossed the species barrier.

Sources of infection

- Exposure in laboratories where the virus is stored.
- Exposure from animal reservoirs (masked palm civet, raccoon dog, Chinese ferret badger).

Natural history

- Affects adults more often than children.
- Incubation period is 2–10 days with a mean of 5 days.
- Present with influenza-like prodromal illness in week 1, with a history of fever.
- By week 2 symptoms of dry cough develop, plus dyspnoea and diarrhoea, with severe cases progressing to respiratory failure.
- Fatality rate of 0–50% varying between countries. Crude global case fatality rate of 9.6%.
- Higher mortality in males and those with comorbidity.

Differential diagnosis of SARS

- Common respiratory pathogens.
  - Predominantly atypical respiratory pathogens, including influenza and parainfluenza, RSV, *Haemophilus*, *Mycoplasma*, *Chlamydia*, *Legionella*, and *Coxiella*.
- Avian influenza.

Radiology

Radiological changes are seen within 3–4 days of the illness. Patchy consolidation or ground glass changes are the most common features. Later features can include pneumothoraces, cystic changes, and subpleural fibrosis.

Laboratory findings

- FBC: lymphopaenia, occasionally thrombocytopaenia.
- Raised LDH.
- Raised ALT/AST.
- Raised CK.
- Occasionally low sodium, potassium, magnesium, and calcium may be seen.

Clinical diagnosis of SARS

History of fever or a documented fever >38°C.

AND

One or more of cough, shortness of breath, or difficulty in breathing.

AND

Radiographic evidence (or autopsy evidence) of lung infiltrates consistent with pneumonia or ARDS.

AND

No more likely alternative diagnosis.

Laboratory diagnosis of SARS

- Positive reverse transcription PCR for SARS coronavirus from:
  - two different clinical specimens.
  - OR two or more sequential specimens.
- Seroconversion by ELISA or IFA:
  - Negative antibody in acute serum with positive convalescent serum.
  - >4-fold rise in antibody level between acute and convalescent serum.
- Viral isolation in cell culture.

Management of suspected case of SARS

- Isolate the patient. Ideally negative-pressure room but at minimum single room. Use masks, gloves, gowns, and goggles.
- Take a thorough history
  - Travel history.
  - History of hospitalization.
  - History of contact with a known case of SARS or laboratory worker with potential contact with SARS.
  - History of contact with a person with fever from an area with SARS.
- Inform the on-call microbiologist.
- Observations and examination concentrating on temperature, pulse oximetry, and respiratory signs.
- Clinical work-up:
  - FBC.
  - U&E, LFT, LDH, CK.
  - Blood cultures.
  - CXR.
  - Sputum for microscopy and culture.
  - Atypical respiratory serology.
  - *Legionella* and pneumoccocal antigen.
  - Serology to save.
- Send samples for diagnostic laboratory tests for coronavirus.
- Treat with broad-spectrum IV antibiotics as per community-acquired pneumonia guidelines until diagnosis confirmed.
- Supportive care.

Currently there is no specific antiviral treatment for SARS. Many centres have used combinations of known antivirals such as ribavirin, some in combination with steroids, but the most effective treatment is unknown. Currently there is no vaccine available for SARS.

Further information

www.who.int/csr/sars

Pleural effusion

ⓘ Introduction

Pleural effusions are a common clinical scenario with a wide range of causes. They are defined as an accumulation of fluid between the visceral and parietal pleura. There is normally around 20 ml of fluid present in the pleural space. Around 400 ml needs to be present before clinically apparent, whilst >200 ml is visible on the PA chest radiograph.

Causes

Divided according to the biochemical characteristics of the fluid into transudate and exudate (see diagnostic investigations below). Although common transudative causes usually result in bilateral effusions, they may result in a unilateral effusion.

Transudate (protein <30 g/L)

Common
- Left ventricular failure.
- Liver cirrhosis.
- Hypoalbuminaemia (e.g. nephrotic syndrome).

Less common
- Pulmonary embolus.
- Hypothyroidism.
- Malignancy (5% are transudative).
- Mitral stenosis.

Exudate (protein >30 g/L)

Common
- Parapneumonic effusion/empyema.
- Pulmonary embolus + infarction.
- Malignancy (often secondary or mesothelioma).
- Tuberculosis.
- Trauma (haemothorax).

Less common
- Connective tissue disease (rheumatoid, SLE).
- Pancreatitis.
- Oesophageal rupture.
- Drugs.
- Chylothorax.

Clinical approach

Thorough history and examination will guide further investigation. A combination of history and examination has been shown to reliably identify transudative causes, obviating the need for immediate diagnostic thoracentesis in some cases.

Symptoms

Ask about:

- Dyspnoea
  - Common even in small effusions.
  - Due to reduced chest wall compliance and lung compression.
  - Often little shunting/hypoxia.
- Chest pain
  - Involvement of parietal pleural or chest wall.
  - Often signifies exudative cause.
  - Pleuritic pain in 75% of PE effusions.
- Cough
  - May be non-specific.
  - Often purulent sputum in empyema.
- Fever
  - Empyema/parapneumonic effusion.
  - TB.
  - Malignancy (mesothelioma/lymphoma).
- Constitutional
  - Weight loss, anorexia + malaise.
  - Seen in TB/empyema/malignancy.
- Skin/eyes/joints
  - Consider rheumatological cause.
- Past medical history
  - Known cardiac disease.
  - Known liver disease.
  - Known renal disease.
  - Oesophageal disease/intervention.
  - History of trauma/rib fractures.
- Drug history
  - Large numbers of drugs can cause an effusion: commonly used include amiodarone, phenytoin, nitrofurantoin, methotrexate.
  - Consult www.pneumotox.com
- Risk factors
  - Exposure to asbestos.
  - Ethnicity and living conditions (TB).
  - Smoking history (malignancy).
  - Risk stratify for embolic disease.

Examination

Features of effusion

- RR and SaO_2 (may be maintained even in moderate effusion).
- Decreased expansion.
- Stony dullness to percussion.
- Decreased breath sounds/vocal resonance.
- Tracheal/mediastinal shift away if large effusion.
- Large effusion with no mediastinal shift: implies associated lung collapse (bronchial carcinoma) or encasement (mesothelioma).

Features of cause

- Basal crackles, raised JVP, peripheral oedema, S3 (CCF).
- Signs of chronic liver disease.
- Facial and peripheral oedema (nephrotic syndrome).
- Hypoxaemia and tachypnoea despite small effusion (consider PE).
- Pyrexia, unwell, hypotension (empyema).
- Cachexia, lymphadenopathy (malignancy, empyema, TB).
- Arthropathy, rash, eye disease (rheumatological).

Investigations

Bloods

- FBC (anaemia, leucocytosis).
- Inflammatory markers (empyema, TB, autoimmune).
- Biochemistry (renal disease, cirrhosis, hypoalbuminaemia).
- Serum total protein, LDH, glucose (paired samples for pleural fluid, see below).
- Clotting (if further intervention is likely, e.g. pleural biopsy, drain insertion).
- Autoantibodies if indicated.
- Serum BNP (if diagnostic doubt about heart failure).

Chest X-ray

- Is the fluid unilateral or bilateral?
- An effusion is normally identified by dependent opacity of the hemithorax with a lateral meniscus.
- Loculated effusions may appear as a rim of lateral shadowing, or as a discrete mass as fluid is encysted within the fissure.
- In the setting of a supine patient (e.g. ICU + ventilated) effusion may appear as a hazy opacification of a hemithorax or thickening of the fissure.
- Look for clues to aetiology (rib fractures, consolidation, lymphadenopathy, discrete mass).

Pleural fluid

When to conduct a diagnostic thoracocentesis?

Pleural fluid analysis is the key to making a precise diagnosis and guides further investigation and management. All pleural effusions of unknown cause should be sampled, except where a transudative cause is diagnosed clinically (e.g. bilateral effusions in clinical context of left ventricular failure).

Current guidelines recommend using a 50 ml syringe with a 21G needle under sterile conditions (📖 Chapter 51).

If the effusion is small or has atypical features on the CXR (e.g. loculations), radiological guidance is required (usually with USS).

If the first attempt at fluid aspiration by a clinician with experience in pleural aspiration is unsuccessful ('dry tap'), further imaging is required. Repeated attempts are potentially dangerous and painful for the patient.

Pleural fluid appearance

- Commonly clear and straw coloured in transudates and some exudates.
- Frank pus
  - Diagnoses empyema.
  - Immediate action required (intercostal drainage, antibiotics).
- Turbid
  - Consider empyema or chylothorax.
- Bloodstained
  - Malignancy/infarction/trauma.
  - True haemothorax will quickly clot in the sampling tube.
  - If in doubt, pleural fluid haematocrit >50% serum haemtocrit is diagnostic of haemothorax.
- Food particles
  - Diagnostic of oesophageal rupture.
  - Immediate action required.

Biochemistry

Immediately send fluid for:
- Protein
- LDH
- Glucose
- pH (via blood gas analyser) ⎫ Assess metabolic activity

Transudate versus exudate

A protein level <25 g/L is a definite transudate and >35 g/L a definite exudate. Between 25 and 35 g/L, or if the serum protein level is abnormal, further assessment is required using Light's criteria:
- pleural fluid protein to serum ratio >0.5.
- pleural fluid LDH to serum ratio >0.6.
- pleural fluid LDH > two-thirds upper limit of normal serum range.

One or more of these criteria is reliably diagnostic of an exudative effusion.

Pleural fluid pH

- Used in the diagnosis of complicated parapneumonic effusion requiring drainage (<7.2).
- Local anaesthetics are acidic and will change the measured value.
- Low pH also seen in malignancy, TB, oesophageal rupture, connective tissue disease.
- Analysis should be by blood gas machine: litmus paper in the laboratory is inaccurate.

Pleural fluid glucose

- Mirrors pleural fluid pH and can be used if pH not available.
- Normally follows serum glucose.
- Low (<1 mmol/L) in empyema, TB, rheumatoid effusion.

Microbiology

The presence of bacteria in the pleural space is always abnormal and diagnostic of pleural infection, even in the absence of biochemical criteria. A sample should be sent for:

- Gram stain.
- Culture + sensitivity.
- Acid-alcohol fast bacilli.
- TB culture (takes up to 9 weeks).

Cell count + cytology

Cell count

May aid in narrowing the differential diagnosis:

- Neutrophil predominant (>50%): suggests an acute process.
- Eosinophilic (>10%): non-specific, may imply air or blood in the pleural space.
- Lymphocyte predominant (>50%): TB + malignancy.

Cytology

- Diagnostic of malignancy in 60% of cases.
- Yield may be increased by a second diagnostic tap.

Special tests

- Pleural fluid amylase should be requested in suspected oesophageal rupture or pancreatitis. Isoenzyme analysis will confirm oesophageal rupture (amylase of salivary origin).
- Autoantibodies should in general not be requested in pleural fluid as they reflect serum levels and add little information.
- In suspected chylothorax (interruption of the thoracic duct leading to chyle leak into the pleural space) pleural fluid triglycerides and cholesterol should be requested (raised triglycerides and normal cholesterol).

Further radiology

Thoracic ultrasound (USS)

- USS is more sensitive in detecting pleural fluid than CXR and allows confirmation of the presence of septations and locules.
- In the case of unsuccessful aspiration or atypical CXR appearances, USS should be requested.
- USS guided aspiration is successful in 97% of cases.

Thoracic CT scan

- If the above tests on pleural fluid are non-diagnostic (e.g. exudate of unknown cause), thoracic CT is the investigation of choice.
- Performed before drainage of effusion and with IV contrast to enable visualization of pleural abnormalities.
- CT is valuable in the diagnosis of malignant and infective pleural disease, and reliably differentiates lung abscess from empyema.

Further tests

- Pleural biopsy ('blind', image guided, or thoracoscopic) may be required: specialist referral is recommended.
- Bronchoscopy has no role in the investigation of pleural effusion, unless an endobronchial lesion associated with collapse is suspected.

Management

Transudates

- Successful management of the underlying disease process will usually result in resolution of the pleural effusion, without recourse to intercostal drainage or further interventions.
- Therapeutic thoracocentesis may be required for short-term symptomatic relief. Removal of as little as 300 ml of fluid (even from a large effusion) may decompress the effusion and ameliorate symptoms.

Exudates

Management depends on cause.
- Traumatic haemothorax: guidelines suggest insertion of a large bore (>18F) chest drain and the space drained to dryness.
- Pleural infection: requires prompt chest drain insertion and antibiotic therapy.
- Oesophageal rupture: associated with a risk of mediastinitis and pleural infection. Patient should be nil by mouth, and a surgical/gastroenterological opinion sought.
- The undiagnosed effusion: if, despite investigation, the cause of effusion remains obscure, TB and PE should be considered (specific therapy available).

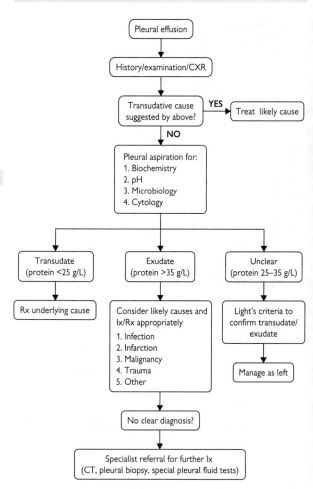

Fig. 24.1 Algorithm for investigation of pleural effusion. (Maskell NA *et al.* (2003). BTS guidelines for the investigation of a unilateral pleural effusion in adults. *Thorax*, **58** (Suppl II), ii8–ii17.)

Pleural infection

① Introduction

A pleural effusion occurs in up to 40% of cases of pneumonia. The majority of these will resolve with treatment of the pneumonia, but a subset will undergo bacterial invasion and subsequent infection will be established. This condition has a high mortality (20%) and morbidity, with 20% of cases requiring invasive thoracic surgery. Early recognition and prompt treatment is important to prevent progression to disease only amenable to surgical treatment.

Some cases of pleural infection are not associated with an underlying pneumonia, most notably iatrogenic and traumatic aetiologies.

Definitions

Parapneumonic effusion (PPE)

Effusion in the context of pneumonia:
- Simple PPE: effusion with no biochemical or microbiological evidence of bacterial invasion.
- Complicated PPE: effusion with biochemical evidence of bacterial invasion.

Empyema

Frank pus in the pleural space.

Pleural infection

Effusion with microbiological evidence of bacterial invasion (even if no biochemical parameters consistent with bacterial invasion).

Pathophysiology

Pleural infection develops as a result of host response to inflammation and bacterial invasion:
- Bacterial infection of the lung is established with associated inflammation and cytokine production.
- Inflammation at the visceral pleural surface results in increased capillary permeability and the formation of fluid within the pleural space (exudative stage = simple PPE).
- Bacteria invade the pleural space, resulting in biochemical changes (complicated PPE). Septations and loculations form.
- Infection is established leading to the production of frank pus (empyema, a combination of dead organisms and leukocytes).
- If infection persists, fibrosis occurs with the formation of a chronically infected thick 'peel' over the visceral and parietal pleura.

Acute presentation

History

- Pleuritic pain is common but not universal.
- Sweats and fevers.
- Weight loss and anorexia.
- Symptoms may be present for a few days or several months.
- History of previous transthoracic procedures, chest trauma or upper GI surgery/interventional endoscopy.

Risk factors

- Diabetes mellitus.
- Alcohol abuse.
- Intravenous drug use.
- Gastro-oesophageal reflux disease.

Examination

- Fever (not universal).
- Tachypnoea, sweaty.
- Cachexia if long history.
- Signs of pleural effusion may be present (may be difficult to detect clinically if loculated collection).

Other presentations

- Pneumonia not resolving on treatment: request repeat/further radiology to assess for the presence of pleural fluid.
- Patients with weight loss, anorexia, fevers, and an abnormal CXR (often mistaken for malignancy): more commonly caused by anaerobic organisms.
- After oesophageal instrumentation/surgery, spontaneous oesophageal perforation (Boerhaeve's syndrome).
- After previous chest drain insertion/pleural procedure (e.g. pneumothorax, drainage of malignant effusion).

Investigations

- Bloods.
- Raised white cell count, CRP, ESR.
- Anaemia of chronic disease, if long history.

Chest radiograph

- May reveal typical features of a small, moderate, or large effusion.
- The presence of pleural fluid in a non-dependent area on the CXR (e.g. lateral collection) makes empyema more likely.
- May present as enlarging mass (encysted fluid in fissure).
- Loculated posterior collections may not be readily identified as pleural fluid.
- Raised hemidiaphragm may be associated with underlying lung collapse, and is difficult to appreciate with effusion present.

CT chest

Request if atypical features as above on the chest radiograph.

- Defines 3D anatomy of the pleural space.
- May identify loculations.
- Permits image-guided catheter insertion.
- Reliably differentiates pulmonary abscess from pleural infection.

Pleural fluid sampling + analysis

When to sample pleural fluid?

- All patients with an effusion in the context of pneumonia, a febrile illness, or recent chest trauma/instrumentation require pleural fluid sampling. This is the key diagnostic step and the results alter immediate management.
- There are no clinical parameters permitting prediction of which parapneumonic effusions require chest tube drainage. Therefore pleural fluid parameters (see later) are the only reliable guide to determine which patients require chest tube drainage.

Key points

- 'Blind' aspiration is often unsuccessful in pleural infection because of the presence of loculations/septations within the fluid, or thickened parietal pleura.
- 'Blind' aspiration should not be attempted, except in cases where radiology and clinical examination are consistent and show a collection of at least moderate size.
- If initial 'blind' attempts are unsuccessful, an image-guided aspiration (normally USS) should be requested on the same day.

Assess pleural fluid for

- Appearance (frank pus/turbid fluid = empyema).
- Pleural fluid pH via blood gas analyser.
- Gram stain, culture, and sensitivity.
- Protein/glucose/LDH.
- Cytology including cell count.

Pleural fluid pH

This investigation differentiates simple from complicated PPE and therefore guides which pleural collections require drainage. pH should not be requested on frankly purulent fluid (may damage blood gas analysers and the result will not alter management). Studies suggest that those PPEs with a lower pH (<7.2) run a more 'complicated' course, requiring chest drainage ± surgical intervention for resolution.

- Pleural fluid pH <7.2 diagnoses complicated PPE; indicates the need for prompt chest tube drainage.
- Not every effusion with a low pH is a complicated PPE (other causes include malignancy, TB, rheumatoid); the context must be considered.
- Not every pleural effusion with a pH >7.2 will run a 'simple' course. Regular review is required and if there is lack of clinical improvement or worsening, a repeat pH sample is advised.

- It is sometimes necessary to institute chest tube drainage in a normal pH effusion (i.e. simple PPE) if this is causing respiratory embarrassment.
- If pH is not available, low pleural fluid glucose (<2.2 mmol/L) is almost as reliable in the selection of those requiring chest tube drainage.

Pleural fluid biochemistry

PPE begins as an exudate (as defined before) but during the simple PPE stage the biochemical characteristics are normal. As bacterial invasion occurs, biochemical changes occur to produce

- low glucose (<2.2 mmol/L)
- high LDH (>1000 IU/L)
- low pH (<7.2)

because of a combination of high metabolic activity, rapid cell turnover and lactate production.

Pleural fluid microbiology

Essential to send a sample for microbiology as soon as possible.

- Combined Gram stain and culture is only positive in around 60% of cases; hence empirical antibiotics required.
- Blood cultures are positive in 12% of cases and should be conducted in all suspected cases (may be the only positive culture).

Microbiology

The microbiology of pleural infection is varied and there are substantial differences between hospital and community-acquired disease. The organisms represent a wider range of pathogens than that seen in pneumonia, with a number of organisms resistant to 'standard' antibiotics for pneumonia.

Most common community-acquired organisms

- Streptococcus milleri.
- Streptococcus pneumoniae.
- Anaerobes.
- Staphylococci.

Most common hospital-acquired organisms

- MRSA (up to one-third of cases).
- Staphylococci.
- Gram-negative bacteria (e.g. Enterobacter).
- Pseudomonas.
- Anaerobes.

Management

Antibiotic therapy
- All patients with suspected pleural infection should receive broad-spectrum antibiotics.
- Empirical therapy is required initially until culture results available. In 40%, no organism is found; thus empirical antibiotics are required for the entire treatment course.
- Do not delay initiating antibiotics whilst waiting for culture results. Start as soon as diagnosis established clinically and cultures taken.
- Antibiotics should be rationalized in the light of positive culture results.
- The optimal length of antibiotic therapy is not known. Most authorities treat for a total of around 3 weeks (with IV therapy over the first 5–7 days).

Empirical antibiotic regimens
Antibiotic choices will be governed by local microbiology and local practice. Suggested empirical regimens are given below, providing broad-spectrum cover for possible organisms.

Community-acquired infection
- Second-generation cephalosporin (e.g. cefuroxime) + anaerobic cover (e.g. metronidazole).
- If penicillin allergic, meropenem 1 g tds IV + metronidazole (po 400 mg tds or IV 500 mg tds).
- Oral treatment: amoxicillin + clavulanic acid (co-amoxiclav).
- In cases of suspected *Legionella*, a macrolide should be added.

Hospital-acquired infection
- Cover required for MRSA, Gram-negative organisms and anaerobes, e.g. meropenem 1 g tds IV + vancomycin 1 g bd IV.
- Oral treatment is not appropriate.

Chest tube drainage
Initiate drainage according to algorithm. Intercostal drainage is required for:
- Empyema (pus/turbid fluid).
- Microbiologically proven infection (pleural Gram stain or culture positive).
- Complicated PPE (pH < 7.2).

Chest drain size
- Small (10–14F) and large (24F+) chest drains may be used.
- Although some authorities recommend large chest drains in the presence of purulent fluid, there are no robust data on which to base decisions about chest drain size in pleural infection.
- If smaller drains are used, regular flushes (e.g. sterile saline 20 ml qds) are recommended.

Radiologically guided drains

- Image-guided drain insertion is often required given the complexities of pleural space anatomy, loculated/septated fluid, and encysted collections seen in pleural infection.
- A low threshold for referral for image-guided drainage is recommended in cases of failed drain insertion at the bedside.

Intrapleural therapy

Previous studies suggested that agents able to lyse septations (thrombolytics) may facilitate chest tube drainage. The largest randomized trial to date suggests no benefit from their use. Therefore intrapleural agents are not recommended on the basis of current evidence.

Drain management

- If drainage stops in the absence of CXR resolution or improved clinical state of the patient, further imaging is recommended to assess drain position.
- Drain repositioning/reinsertion may be required.

Further management

- Patients with pleural infection should be under the care of a respiratory physician.
- Further management options are surgical and require specialist referral.

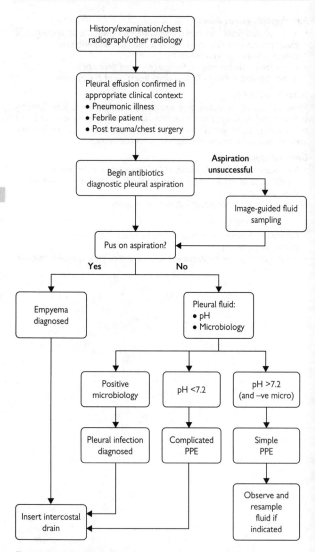

Fig. 25.1 Algorithm for diagnosis/early management of pleural infection.
(Davies CW (2003). BTS guidelines for the management of pleural infection.
Thorax **58** (Suppl II), ii18–ii28.)

Pneumothorax

Definitions

Pneumothorax is defined as air in the pleural space. It may occur as a result of trauma or spontaneously, in which case it is further subdivided into primary and secondary. The treatment, response to therapy, and prognosis in these two groups is quite different, and establishing the category is essential.

Any pneumothorax may result in a tension pneumothorax, which requires immediate intervention to prevent rapid deterioration and potentially death. There remains significant mortality from all causes of pneumothorax.

Primary spontaneous pneumothorax (PSP)

PSP has an incidence of 18–28 in 100 000 per year for men and 16.7 in 100 000 per year for women. Most common in men aged 20–40 years.

Pathophysiology

Although PSP occurs in otherwise healthy lungs, small areas of abnormally dilated air spaces (subpleural blebs and bullae) are commonly found in apical areas of lung where pneumothorax has occurred. These areas are thought to rupture, leading to air escaping from the lung into the pleural space.

Risk factors

- Smoking: lifetime risk in smoking men of 12% versus 0.1% in non-smokers.
- Tall stature: greater pressure at apical blebs.

Prognosis

- Risk of recurrence after first episode of PSP is around 30% over 2 years, increasing to 40% and 50% after second and third episodes, respectively.
- Continued smoking increases the risk of recurrence (directly related to amount smoked), up to 100× in some studies of heavy smokers.
- PSP has a very low mortality in the absence of tension pneumothorax (in contrast with secondary pneumothorax).

Secondary spontaneous pneumothorax (SSP)

Associated with:

- COPD (most cases).
- Asthma.
- Fibrotic lung disease.
- TB.

- Cystic fibrosis.
- Marfan's syndrome.
- Lung carcinoma (peripheral).
- Pneumocystis pneumonia.

Prognosis

- Risk of recurrence: 40–80% depending on underlying lung disease.
- Large air leaks more common with associated complications.
- Mortality 10%: therefore aggressive management.

✚ Acute presentation

Initial questions

- Any evidence of tension pneumothorax (see below)? If so, manage immediately.
- Is the patient truly breathless (not just shallow breathing due to pleuritic pain)?
- Is there evidence of underlying lung disease?

History

- Chest pain: sudden onset, often pleuritic and usually preceding other symptoms (thought to be secondary to ripping of adhesions between visceral and parietal pleura).
- Breathlessness: sudden onset. May not be present in small pneumothoraces (especially primary) but may be severe and present as an acute on chronic exacerbation (e.g. COPD).
- Duration of symptoms: almost 50% of patients have symptoms of pneumothorax for 2 days before presenting. A long history should not put you off the diagnosis, and may be associated with re-expansion pulmonary oedema.
- Previous history of lung disease and chronic respiratory symptoms.
- Previous episodes and previous treatments.
- Previous history of trauma (may present some time after traumatic event): consider traumatic pneumothorax. Occurs secondary to penetrating chest trauma (includes rib fracture), deceleration injury of the lung and/or increased intrathoracic pressure (e.g. blunt chest trauma) leading to alveolar rupture.
- Consider iatrogenic pneumothorax after the following:
  - Chest aspiration.
  - Subclavian central line insertion.
  - Transbronchial biopsy at bronchoscopy.
  - Image-guided lung biopsy.
  - Positive pressure ventilation (may occur in the absence of chest instrumentation/trauma).
  - Intercostal nerve block.
  - Chest compression (NB post-resuscitation).

Examination

- If tracheal deviation away from the affected side and shocked patient (low blood pressure, tachycardia, cardiovascular collapse), tension pneumothorax has occurred and requires immediate action (see below).
- Decreased breath sounds, decreased expansion, and hyper-resonance of the affected side.

☠ Tension pneumothorax

This is a medical emergency: do not request further investigations (e.g CXR)

- Occurs due to a one-way valve in the visceral pleura allowing air from the lung into the pleural space with each inspiration, progressively increasing pleural pressure.
- Increased pleural pressure causes mediastinal shift and diaphragm inversion, eventually resulting in compromised right ventricular filling, cardiovascular collapse, and EMD arrest.
- May occur in pneumothoraces of any size.
- High suspicion in patients on positive pressure ventilation (including non-invasive ventilation).

The patient

- Agitation, respiratory distress.
- Hypotension, tachycardia, weak pulse.
- Raised JVP, tracheal deviation.
- Decreased expansion and breath sounds on affected side.
- EMD arrest.

Immediate management

- High-flow oxygen.
- Decompress the hemithorax
  - Insert large bore cannula (at least 4.5 cm long) into second intercostal space in mid-clavicular line on the side of signs.
  - Hiss of air on entering the pleural space confirms diagnosis.
  - Aspirate until patient stable (relief may occur only a few seconds after initial hiss).
  - Note: almost two-thirds of patients have chest walls thicker than 3 cm. Therefore a cannula at least 4.5 cm long is recommended.
- Definitive management: leave cannula in place as definitive intercostal drain is placed (should not be placed anteriorly; place in mid-axillary line).

Investigations

CXR

Diagnostic in most cases. Look for:

- Thin shadow of the lung edge and absent lung markings peripherally.
- Blunting of costophrenic angle on side of pneumothorax (small effusion due to bleed).
- Evidence of developing tension (deviated trachea, mediastinal shift, depressed hemidiaphragm).
- Evidence of underlying lung disease.

Size classification

Current guidelines take into account volume estimations from a 2D image (i.e. the CXR):

- <2 cm rim of pneumothorax from chest wall = small
- >2 cm rim of pneumothorax from chest wall = large

Note

- A >2 cm rim approximates to a 50% pneumothorax by volume. This size classification determines management.
- Marked breathlessness in a patient with <2 cm pneumothorax may herald the development of tension.

Pitfalls

- Substantial subcutaneous emphysema.
- Differentiating between a large bulla and a pneumothorax.
- On supine CXR, pneumothoraces may only manifest as increased lucency of the chest ± sharply delineated heart border.
- Very small pneumothoraces are reliably detected by a lateral decubitus CXR.

CT chest

Considered the gold standard for diagnosis of even tiny pneumothoraces. Also recommended in cases where subcutaneous emphysema obscures the chest radiograph and for the differentiation of bullae and pneumothoraces. Used in cases of high-impact trauma to detect unsuspected pneumothorax.

ABGs

Not a required investigation in every case. Majority will show evidence of hypoxia, with hypercapnia associated with underlying lung disease.

:O: Management

Authorities and guidelines differ in management of pneumothorax. The following is based on the British Thoracic Society Guidelines 2003 (see Figs 26.1 and 26.2).

Management is based on:
- The degree of breathlessness.
- The presence of underlying lung disease.
- The size of pneumothorax.

Observation

- PSP: no intervention required where the rim is <2 cm and the patient is not breathless.
- Observation is not recommended for SSP or for any patient with breathlessness regardless of the size of pneumothorax. These patients will need intervention (see below).
- Early outpatient review must be in place if discharged.

Oxygen

High-flow O_2 should be used during admissions in appropriate patients (non-CO_2 retainers). This increases the reabsorption rate of the pneumothorax.

Aspiration

📖 Chapter 51 for practical procedure.
- PSP: aspiration is recommended as first line for all pneumothoraces requiring intervention (60–80% success rate). A second aspiration should be considered if the first is unsuccessful (30% success rate).
- SSP: aspiration is less successful (30–60%) and is not recommended except where:
  - the rim is <2 cm
  - the patient is <50 years old.

After successful aspiration a period of in-hospital observation (24 hours) is required.
- Aspiration should be stopped if substantial pain or cough occurs or if >2.5 L of air is aspirated (implies ongoing air leak).
- Newer treatments: catheter aspiration of simple pneumothorax (CASP) involves passing an 8F catheter which can be repeatedly aspirated and easily removed. Ambulatory treatment is sometimes used with Heimlich or flutter valves.

Intercostal drainage + complications

📖 Chapter 52 for practical procedure.
- The majority of PSPs do not require intercostal drainage.
- Drainage is associated with a significant rate of morbidity (incorrect placement, infection, bleeding).
- First-line treatment for large SSPs or after failed aspiration.
- Smaller (10–14F) tubes are usually adequate; larger (>24F) tubes may be required (air leak or subcutaneous emphysema).

- Never clamp a bubbling chest drain (conversion to tension).
- Persistent air leak: use of clamping and suction should be referred to a specialist.

Post-treatment advice

- Patients with a current pneumothorax must not fly. After radiologically proven resolution, they may fly within 2 weeks.
- After any pneumothorax, the patient may NEVER dive (using compressed air) unless a definitive surgical treatment is conducted.

① Complications

Re-expansion pulmonary oedema

May occur as a complication of treatment for pneumothorax (up to 14%), especially in PSP present for some time before treatment. Higher incidence in large pneumothoraces and younger patients. Mechanism unknown, but may be related to capillary damage and leak in the re-expanding lung.

Clinical manifestations

- Cough
- Breathlessness　⎫ After drain insertion
- Chest tightness　⎭

Management

- Observation: usually resolves within 24–48 hours.
- Avoid suction early in the treatment of PSP.

Surgical/subcutaneous emphysema

Definition

Air escaping into the subcutaneous tissues from a pneumothorax.

Mechanism

Air escapes under pleural pressure via a connection between the pneumothorax and the subcutaneous tissues, usually a complication of chest drain insertion. May occur if:

- Chest drain is non-functioning (kinked, malpositioned, clamped).
- Large air leak (insufficient drainage, especially COPD).

The patient

- Feel for 'crackles' as you compress the skin.
- Usually occurs around drain insertion site initially but may track to arms, face, and contralateral chest wall.
- Occasionally may be life-threatening (respiratory compromise due to upper airway compression). Look for facial involvement and/or voice change (laryngeal emphysema).

Management

Normally self-resolving and of cosmetic importance only. High-flow oxygen (increases rate of resolution) can be used unless the patient is known to retain CO_2. If evidence of upper airway involvement:

- Specialist referral as soon as possible.
- High flow oxygen.
- Second/larger bore chest drain.
- Skin incisions ("blow holes") and push air out by massaging the skin.

Tracheostomy is rarely required.

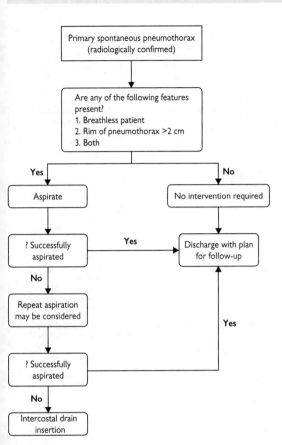

Fig. 26.1 Algorithm for management of primary pneumothorax. (Henry M *et al.* (2003). BTS guidelines for the management of spontaneous pneumothorax. *Thorax*, **58** (Suppl II), ii39–ii52.)

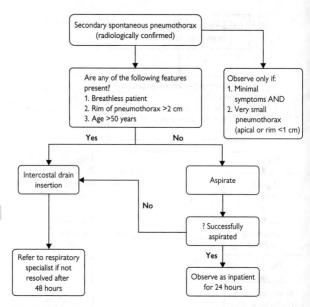

Fig. 26.2 Algorithm for management of secondary pneumothorax. (Henry M et al. (2003). BTS guidelines for the management of spontaneous pneumothorax. *Thorax*, **58** (Suppl II), ii39–ii52.)

Pneumonia

① Pneumonia

Pneumonia is a commonly used term in both medical practice and the community at large. It is often used synonymously (and erroneously) with terms such as 'chest infection', 'bronchitis', or 'infective exacerbation of COPD'. It is subdivided into several different entities reflecting the different epidemiology, presentation, bacteriology, and therapy required.

Community-acquired pneumonia

The definition of community-acquired pneumonia (CAP) in the hospital setting is as follows.

- Symptoms and signs consistent with an acute lower respiratory tract infection associated with new radiographic shadowing for which there is no other explanation (e.g. not pulmonary oedema or infarction).
- Symptoms and signs occur at presentation or within 48 hours of hospital admission.

Epidemiology

- Annual incidence in the community is 5–11 in 1000 adults.
- Between 22% and 42% of adults with CAP are admitted to hospital.
- Between 5% and 10% of adults admitted with CAP are managed on ICU.
- Mortality in those admitted to hospital is reported to be 5–12%.
- Mortality in those admitted to UK ICUs is as high as 50%.

Risks

- Alcoholism.
- Chronic cardiorespiratory disease.
- Diabetes.
- Elderly.
- Oral corticosteroids or other immunosuppression, in whom typical features may be absent.

Bacteriology

The causative agent cannot be accurately predicted from the clinical, laboratory, or radiographic data available. No pathogen is isolated in approximately 40–70% of cases in routine clinical practice. Potential organisms include the following.

- *Streptococcus pneumoniae*: most common pathogen in CAP.
- *Haemophilus influenzae*: common in acute exacerbations of COPD.
- *Staphylococcus aureus*: often following viral infection.
- *Moraxella catarrhalis*.
- Gram-negative bacteria, e.g. *Klebsiella*, *Pseudomonas*.
- Anaerobic bacteria.
- *Mycoplasma pneumoniae*: occurs in 4-yearly cycles.
- *Legionella pneumophilia*: common in severe CAP.
- *Chlamydia pneumoniae* and *Chlamydia psittaci* (psittacosis).
- Influenza A and B.

Investigations

📖 Chapter 5.

Severity assessment

Once pneumonia is diagnosed the assessment of severity forms a key part of effective patient care. Poor prognosis is indicated by:

- Increasing age.
- Coexisting disease.
- Absence of fever.
- Elevated respiratory rate.
- Confusion.
- Elevated blood urea.
- Hypotension and tissue hypoperfusion (↑lactate).
- Hypoxaemia.
- WCC <4 or >20 × 10^9/L.
- Bilateral radiographic infiltrates.
- Positive blood cultures.

The CURB-65 score is a validated method of assessing the severity and prognosis of community-acquired pneumonia. It is simple to perform and should be done routinely as part of the admission procedure. It consists of five points.

- Confusion: new disorientation in time, place, and person or an abbreviated mental test score ≤8.
- Urea >7 mmol/L.
- Respiratory rate >30 breaths/minute.
- Blood pressure: DBP <60 mmHg or SBP <90 mmHg.
- Age >65 years.

CURB-65 score

- 0–1: low risk of death, has non-severe pneumonia, and may be suitable for outpatient care.
- 2: recommend a short hospital stay and IV antibiotics.
- >3: patient at high risk of death and should be treated as severe pneumonia in hospital.
- ≥4: critical care involvement should be considered.

Antibiotic therapy

The choice of initial antibiotic is guided by the severity of the pneumonia, the treatment setting, the ability of the patient to take penicillin and local antibiotic sensitivities, and prescribing practices. Current BTS recommendations for empirical therapy in CAP are shown in Table 27.1.

Table 27.1 BTS recommendations for empirical therapy in CAP

Severity of pneumonia	Penicillin sensitive	Penicillin allergic
Non-severe: community treatment	Amoxicillin 500 mg to 1 g tds po	Erythromycin 500 mg qds po or clarithromycin 500 mg bd po
Non-severe: hospital treatment, oral	Amoxicillin 500 mg to 1 g tds po PLUS Eythromycin 500 mg qds po or clarithromycin 500 mg bd po	Erythromycin 500 mg qds po or clarithromycin 500 mg bd po OR Levofloxacin 500 mg od po or moxifloxacin 400 mg od po
Non-severe: hospital treatment, IV therapy	Ampicillin 500 mg qds IV or benzylpenicillin 1.2 g qds IV PLUS Erythromycin 500 mg qds IV or clarithromycin 500 mg bd IV	Fluoroquinolone with enhanced pneumococcal activity, e.g. Levofloxacin 500 mg od po
Severe pneumonia	Co-amoxiclav 1.2 g tds IV or cefuroxime 1.5 g tds IV or ceftriaxone 2 g od IV PLUS Erythromycin 500 mg qds IV or cefotaxime 1 g tds or clarithromycin 500 mg bd IV (± rifampicin 600 mg od)	Fluoroquinolone with enhanced pneumococcal activity, e.g. levofloxacin 500 mg bd IV PLUS benzylpencillin 1.2 g qds IV

Hospital-acquired pneumonia

Hospital-acquired pneumonia (HAP), also known as nosocomial pneumonia, is recognized as pneumonia developing at least 48 hours after hospital admission. It accounts for 10–20% of hospital-acquired infections. Some people use the phrase 'healthcare-associated pneumonia' to encompass both HAP and pneumonia occurring in those living in long-term care environments for whom traditional CAP bacteriology and therapy do not apply. HAP has a poor prognosis, with a mortality of up to 50%. Failure to improve should prompt a search for pleural infection or lung abscess. ICU care should be sought early if appropriate.

Risk factors

Include impaired host defences, impaired conscious levels and aspiration, reduced gastric pH from medications, and broad-spectrum antibiotic usage.

Bacteriology

In contrast with CAP:
- Mixed infection is common.
- Aerobes commonly include *S.aureus* and Gram-negative rods (*Pseudomonas*, *Klebsiella*, coliforms).

- Anaerobes are important pathogens.
- Multiresistant organisms, including MRSA, should always be considered. Antibiotics should be given intravenously initially and cover the above organisms. Possible regimens include:
- Cefuroxime (750–1500 mg tds) and metronidazole (500 mg tds).
- To cover *Pseudomonas* infection consider piperacillin/tazobactam 4.5 g tds, ceftazidime 1–2 g tds, gentamicin 3–5 mg/kg od, or meropenem 500–1000 mg tds.
- Vancomycin 1 g bd or teicoplanin 400 mg od are required to cover MRSA.

Aspiration pneumonia

Occurs due to aspiration of material from the upper airways or GI tract into the lower airways. Risk factors include a reduced level of consciousness, gastro-oesophageal reflux, dysphagia, and recent upper GI surgery. Aspiration may cause a bacterial pneumonia or a chemical pneumonitis.

Bacterial pneumonia

Caused by pathogens which usually inhabit the upper respiratory or GI tract.
- Classically affects the dependent lung segments, e.g. usually right lower lobe or posterior segment right upper lobe on lying flat.
- Antibiotics which include cover of anaerobic organisms are traditional although this is debated by some.
  - Cefuroxime (750–1500 mg) tds and metronidazole (500 mg) tds IV.
  - Co-amoxiclav (1.0 g) tds IV.

Aspiration pneumonitis

The aspiration of substances into the lower airways causing a rapid inflammatory process to develop in the lung. It is not caused by bacteria.
- Care is supportive.
- Antibiotics for pneumonia are often given as it may be hard to separate the two diagnoses and secondary infection of pneumonitis is common.
- Steroids occasionally used with little evidence of benefit.

Ventilator-associated pneumonia

Ventilator-associated pneumonia (VAP) is the combination of symptoms and signs of pneumonia with new consolidation on CXR, developing at least 48 hours after endotracheal intubation. It is thought to be a consequence of repeated aspiration of upper airways secretions into the lower airway. A cuffed endotracheal tube or tracheostomy may reduce aspiration but will not eliminate it. The normal pulmonary clearance mechanisms are then unable to clear the lower airways.
- A respiratory physician may be asked to perform a bronchoscopic BAL to obtain a sample for microbiologic analysis. Some units use a non-directed BAL using a suction catheter to obtain repeated samples.
- Antibiotics are broad spectrum (e.g. meropenem or piperacillin/ tazobactam) to cover HAP and should be discussed with the microbiologist.

Complications/failure to improve

Pleural infection

The presence of either an empyema or complicated parapneumonic effusion implies an infected pleural space and further therapy is indicated.

- Pleural infection should be suspected in any patient with pneumonia who is failing to improve as predicted.
- It should be investigated with CXR, thoracic ultrasound, or CT scanning if atypical features on CXR, and pleural sampling to guide definitive management (📖 Chapter 25).
- If pleural infection is confirmed advice from a respiratory physician should be sought.

Pulmonary abscess

This is necrosis of the lung parenchyma. It is usually the consequence of aspiration pneumonia and therefore the risk factors are the same.

- Classic features include a cough productive of foul sputum if the cavity communicates with an airway. Cavities seen on CXR may have air–fluid levels.
- Pulmonary abscess formation in IV drug users should prompt a search for right heart infective endocarditis.
- *Klebsiella*, *S.aureus*, anaerobes, and TB are the most common bacteria to cause cavitation.
- Empirical antibiotic therapy with cefuroxime 1.5 g tds IV, metronidazole 500 mg tds IV ± flucloxacillin 1 g qds IV.
- Consider radiologically guided percutaneous drainage in those who fail to respond to antibiotics and supportive treatment.

Lemierre's syndrome

- Rare infection of young adults.
- Pharyngitis due to anaerobic bacterium *Fusobacterium necrophorum*.
- Spreads to neck and carotid sheath, causing jugular venous thrombophlebitis and thrombosis.
- Bacteraemia results in septic emboli to other organs including lung.

Further reading

1. Macfarlane JT et al. (2001). BTS guidelines on the management of community acquired pneumonia in adults. *Thorax*, **56** (Suppl 4), 1–64.
2. BTS guidelines for the management of community acquired pneumonia in adults – 2004 update. Available online at: www.brit-thoracic.org.uk/guidelines
3. Bacterial respiratory infection, Chapter 20, OHRM.

Pulmonary embolism

Introduction

Pulmonary embolism (PE) can present with numerous non-specific symptoms and signs and hence mimics several other clinical conditions.

The annual incidence of PE is approximately 60–70 cases in 100 000. Half occur in hospitalized patients, with a quarter having clear risk factors and the remainder being idiopathic. Most hospitals will have their own protocol for investigation; some still use ventilation–perfusion scintigraphy if they have on-site facilities, but most now use multi-detector CT pulmonary angiography (CTPA).

This chapter outlines a practical strategy for the diagnosis and management of PE, including when to suspect it, associated clinical features, the key importance of pre-test probabilities, and the controversies around treatment.

PE is subdivided into massive PE and submassive PE according to the degree of haemodynamic compromise. Massive PE causes a systolic BP <90 mmHg (or fall >40 mmHg) for >15 minutes.

Risk factors

Major risk factors (relative risk 5–20)

- **Surgery:** especially major abdominal/pelvic, hip/knee replacement, post-operative intensive care.
- **Obstetrics:** pregnancy, caesarean section, post-delivery.
- **Lower limb fractures** and varicose veins.
- **Malignancy.**
- **Immobilization:** institutionalization.
- **Previous venous thromboembolism.**

Minor risk factors (relative risk 2–4)

- Cardiovascular: congenital heart disease, CCF, hypertension, superficial thrombophlebitis, indwelling central access.
- Oestrogens: oral contraception and hormone replacement therapy.
- COPD.
- Thrombophilia.
- Long-distance travel.
- Neurological disorders.
- Obesity.
- Chronic disease, e.g. dialysis, vasculitidies especially Behçet's syndrome.

Clinical probability

⚠ Before ordering any specific investigations for PE (including D-dimer) a clinical probability *must* be determined. Essentially all strategies for investigation rely on this, and if it is not consciously done then the pathway to exclusion or confirmation becomes unclear.

Scoring for pre-test probability: British Thoracic Society guidance

- Is a clinical pattern of PE present?
  - Collapse with raised JVP? (Feeling faint or hypotensive).
  - Pulmonary haemorrhage syndrome (pleuritic pain ± haemoptysis).
  - Isolated dyspnoea (no chest pain/cough/sputum).
  If YES ask the following questions:
- Are alternative diagnoses *unlikely* either clinically or with the benefit of white cell count, chest radiograph, ECG, spirometry or peak flow?
  If YES score +1
- Is a major risk factor present?
  - Major surgery or recent immobilization.
  - Recent lower limb trauma or surgery.
  - Clinical DVT.
  - Previous proven DVT/PE.
  - Pregnancy or post-partum.
  - Major medical illness.
  If YES score +1
- Pathway for action;
  - Score +2: **high** probability. Heparinize and investigate urgently.
  - Score +1: **intermediate** probability. Heparinize, early tests for PE but also seek alternative diagnoses.
  - Score 0: **low** probability. Wait for test results, consider investigations, and pursue alternative diagnoses.

Specific investigations once armed with pre-test probability

- High probability
  - D-dimer is not helpful.
  - Proceed to CTPA (or isotope perfusion scan if CXR is normal and no cardiorespiratory disease). If CTPA is good quality and negative then no further investigations are needed.
  - If isotope perfusion scan is non-diagnostic, proceed to CTPA.
  - In patients with coexisting clinical DVT, leg ultrasound as the initial imaging test is usually sufficient.
- Intermediate probability:
  - D-dimer (ELISA test: laboratory-based quantitative assay not latex-based bedside assay). Each laboratory has its own range.
  - If D-dimer above threshold proceed to CTPA (or VQ as above). If D-dimer is below threshold PE is excluded.
- Low probability:
  - D-dimer (agglutination tests, e.g. SimpliRED also acceptable).
  - If above threshold, proceed to CTPA. If below threshold PE is excluded.

☢ **Submassive PE**

▶ When to suspect submassive PE

Symptoms and signs in descending order of frequency from 70%.

- Dyspnoea.
- Tachypnoea.
- Pleuritic pain.
- Apprehension.
- Tachycardia.
- Cough.
- Haemoptysis.
- Leg pain.
- Clinical DVT (in only 10%).

Fever is common but completely non-specific (less likely if >38.9°C).

Examination findings

Tachypnoea and tachycardia should be noted. Occasionally a rub may be heard but these findings are neither sensitive nor specific.

General investigations

ECG

- Most common finding is sinus tachycardia.
- Non-specific ST and T wave changes are common.
- Right heart strain may be seen; the classic $S_1Q_3T_3$ is uncommon, but some features may be noted (Fig. 28.1).

CXR

- Most useful for demonstrating alternative diagnoses.
- Wedge-shaped classical pulmonary infarcts are rare and the oligaemic Westermark's sign is uncommon (☐ Chapter 9).

Other blood tests

- Arterial blood gases may show hypoxia and a raised A–a gradient.
- Raised inflammatory markers may suggest alternative diagnoses.
- D-dimer.
  - D-dimer is a breakdown product of fibrinolysis.
  - D-dimer is sensitive but non specific for the presence of endovascular clot.
  - It is useful for its negative predictive value in low and intermediate probability venous thromboembolism, but has no useful positive predictive value.
  - This means that you should never investigate for a PE if the only finding is a raised D-dimer, as you are exposing the patient to the risks of the investigation.
  - The BTS has produced a statement on the use of the D-dimer assay stressing the importance of proper pre-test assessment (Fig. 28.2).

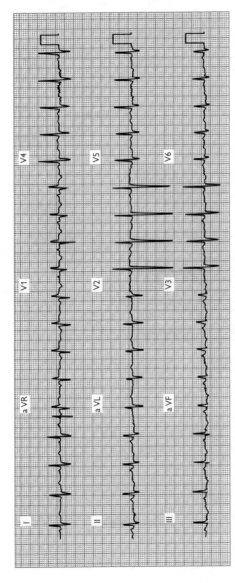

Fig. 28.1 ECG in a patient with multiple large PEs: note the S wave in I, inverted T waves in III, and the positive R in V1. However, there is no Q in lead III.

The advice below is for middle-grade medical staff in A&E

1. Is chest X-ray poor quality? *If so*, arrange departmental PA film ➜

2. Was assessement inadequate? *If so*, review carefully, considering non-PE diagnoses ➜

3. Does PE seem a resonable possibility? *If so*, consult flowchart below ➜

4. Are you unsure whether CTPA is justified? *If so*, LMWH and await consultant decion.

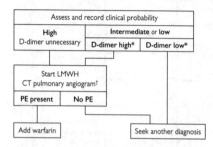

* Refers to *quantitative* tests. Qualitative (+ve/–ve) only useful if low probability, not recommended

† Or V/Q, but only if (a) normal CXR and no chronic cardiorespiratory diseases, of (b) pregnant

For clinical probability (which assumes that PE is a reasonable possibility):

• Is PE more likely than any alternative?	*If so*, score **+1**
• Is there a *major* risk factor for‡ VTE?	*If so*, score **+1**
• Probability form total score is	**2 = high, 1 = intermediate, 0 = low**

‡ Recent immobilty/major surgery/leg fracture, previous, DVT/PE, obstetric, metastatic cancer.
Does not include minor risks: oestrogens, travel, known thrombophilia, obesity, minor surgery.

Fig. 28.2 Use of the D-dimer assay.

Treatment of submassive PE

LMWH should be started as soon as the diagnosis is suspected in high or intermediate probability patients and stopped if tests are negative. It should be withheld in low-risk patients until a D-dimer is available (although if immobile inpatients, consider prophylactic heparin). Dosing is weight based on ranges, exact units, or mg/kg depending upon brand.

Duration of treatment

- For short-term risks (e.g. immediately post-surgery) 4–6 weeks is sufficient.
- For a first idiopathic thrombus 3 months.
- For all others 6 months.
- Long-term anticoagulation is often recommended in recurrent DVT/PE especially without significant risk factors.

Key areas of caution

⚠ Renal failure (creatinine clearance <30ml/kg/minute)

- These patients accumulate LMWH; therefore use unfractionated heparin and seek advice from your local renal team.
- Some centres may use in conjunction with anti-Xa activity monitoring.

⚠ Pregnancy

- D-dimers are likely to be positive (however, are still useful if negative).
- LMWH dose should be given according to actual weight (not pre-pregnancy weight).
- There is evidence that 10–20% higher doses per kg are required.
- Ideally anti-Xa levels should be monitored.
- Switch to unfractionated heparin as delivery date approaches.
- Liaison with experts in obstetric medicine is advisable.

Mechanical options

Some patients are such high risk for anticoagulation that it must be withheld, e.g.

- Pelvic fractures awaiting fixation.
- Recent intracranial or spinal haemorrhage or surgery.

If anticoagulation needs to be withheld for more than 24 hours then mechanical options should be considered in consultation with interventional radiology:

- Clot dispersion or fragmentation using pulmonary artery catheter devices.
- Use of inferior vena caval filters to prevent further embolization. Subsequent anticoagulation will be necessary to prevent filter occlusion and filter removal is possible at a later stage in some patients (if an appropriate filter is used initially).

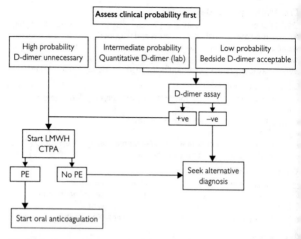

Fig. 28.3 Algorithm for management of submassive PE. Some centres may use VQ scanning initially in those with a normal CXR and no pre-existing pulmonary/cardiac pathology (see BTS Guidelines).

☠ Massive PE

▶▶ When to suspect massive PE

Massive PE is likely if all of the following are present.

- Collapse and/or hypotension.
- Hypoxia without other explanation.
- Engorged neck veins or markedly raised JVP.
- Right ventricular third sound (gallop).

Managing shock in massive PE (📖 Chapter 1)

- High-flow oxygen.
- IV access.
- Analgesia (caution with hypotension).
- ⚠ Fluid load may be helpful but be very cautious beyond 500 ml as it may worsen RV failure and the increased RV wall stress may worsen the perfusion of and hence contractility of the right heart.
- See Fig. 28.4 for use of thrombolysis and heparin.
- If vasopressors are required then small boluses of metaraminol with institution of a noradrenaline infusion are the best option (📖 Chapter 1).
- ⚠ If central access is required make sure it is expert as accidental arterial puncture may prevent the subsequent use of thrombolysis.
- Avoid the subclavian route.
- Once PE has been confirmed, in stable patients give alteplase as 10 mg IV over 1–2 minutes followed by IV infusion of 50 mg over 60 minutes, then 4 infusions each of 10 mg over 30 minutes.
- Thrombolysis should be followed after 3 hours by a weight-adjusted unfractionated heparin infusion.

✦ Treat in hospital or at home?

- There is still some controversy about whether people with PE should be treated in hospital until they are established on oral anticoagulants.
- There is good evidence that they should be treated with parenteral anticoagulation until the warfarin levels are in range (lower rate of recurrent events than if oral anticoagulants alone are used). There is some evidence this should be for a minimum of 5 days.
- The BTS recommends that stable non-compromised patients should be managed as outpatients in the same way as is now done for DVT.

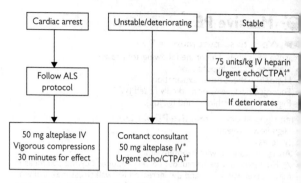

* If thrombolysis contraindicated because of high risk of bleeding, consider radiologically guided clot fragmentation or open thrombectomy if these facilities are available.
† Choice of echo or CTPA will depend upon expertise available and patient stability.

Fig. 28.4 Management algorithm for massive PE.

urther investigation of patients ollowing PE

- Testing for thrombophilia is only indicated if venous thrombo-embolism (VTE) is recurrent (without obvious major risk factors) or in those with VTE and a strong family history.
- If you feel thrombophilia screening might be helpful, discuss the patient with a haematologist before requesting the tests.
- If the patient is known to have a factor deficiency, discuss length of anticoagulation with haematologist.
- Investigations for occult malignancy are only indicated in idiopathic VTE if symptoms, signs or routine investigation raise clinical suspicion.

Prevention of pulmonary emboli

Consider prophylaxis in all inpatients

- Peri-operative prophylaxis is now routine practice in most hospitals.
- Medical patients are also at high risk because of immobility, particularly CCF, COPD, patients with chest drains inserted.
- Half of all PEs occur in hospitalized/institutionalized patients. Of those surviving the initial event, 7% die within 1 week, and 18% by 3 months *despite* standard treatment. Historical figures suggest a mortality of 30% without treatment.
- If chemical prophylaxis is contraindicated, patients should have TED stockings and automatic foot or calf compression pumps.

References and further reading

British Thoracic Society (2003). British Thoracic Society guidelines for the management of suspected acute pulmonary embolism. *Thorax*, **58**, 470–484. Available online at: www.brit-thoracic.org.uk

British Thoracic Society (1997). British Thoracic Society Guidelines *Thorax* **52** (Suppl 4), S2–S24. Available online at: www.brit-thoracic.org.uk

PIOPED Investigators (1990). PIOPED I Study. *JAMA*. **263**, 2753–9.

PIOPED Investigators (2006). PIOPED II Study *N Engl J Med*, **354**, 2317–27.

British Society for Haematology Guidelines: useful guidance on anticoagulation, D-dimers and when to test and treat patients with thrombophilia. Available online at: www.bcshguidelines.com

Pulmonary–renal syndromes

① **Pulmonary–renal syndromes**

The combination of new-onset respiratory signs, symptoms and abnormal investigations together with acute renal dysfunction could indicate a 'pulmonary–renal syndrome'. Whilst renal dysfunction may follow on from systemic illness such as severe sepsis due to pneumonia, the term 'pulmonary–renal syndrome' is by convention taken to mean new alveolar haemorrhage and glomerulonephritis due to a systemic vasculitis.

Vasculitides are amongst the most interesting and challenging conditions which may present to the acute physician. Untreated, they have high mortality rates and therapy requires the use of high doses of immunosuppressant and often single or multi-organ support.

Classification

The pulmonary–renal syndromes are small vessel vasculitides and include the following.

- Wegener's granulomatosis
  - Upper airway problems and a positive c-ANCA/anti-PR3 are highly suggestive of Wegener's granulomatosis.
- Microscopic polyangiitis
  - Can be both c- and p-ANCA positive. Hard to differentiate from Wegener's granulomatosis.

The combination of immunofluoresence and anti-PR3/MPO increases sensitivity and specificity for the diagnosis of Wegener's and microscopic polyangiitis to over 90%.

- Goodpasture's disease.
  - Linear deposition of IgG is seen along the basement membranes of lung and glomeruli. Anti-GBM antibodies can be detected in blood. 'Anti-GBM disease' refers to renal failure due to anti-GBM antibodies without pulmonary involvement.
- Churg–Strauss syndrome.
  - The constellation of asthma, eosinophilic granulomatous airway inflammation, small vessel vasculitis, and peripheral blood eosinophilia >10%. May affect other organs; mononeuritis multiplex is common. p-ANCA is positive in about 60% and lung or sural nerve biopsy should be considered.

History

Vasculitides are difficult to diagnose from the history alone. They should be suspected in patients who have been unwell for several weeks or months with non-specific symptoms. Patients have often been investigated and treated for other diseases. A 'vasculitic screen' will have been done as part of a search for the diagnosis.

Symptoms

- **Upper airway**: epistaxis, nasal congestion, sinusitis, mucosal ulceration, septal perforation, and laryngeal abnormality. In Wegener's granulomatosis upper airway symptoms are commonly the first noticed.
- **Respiratory**: haemoptysis due to small vessel vasculitis and alveolar haemorrhage is the classic symptom. Cough without haemoptysis, dyspnoea, pleuritic pain, and wheeze are also seen.

- **Renal**: frank haematuria is rare; oliguria may be seen as renal failure progresses.
- **Systemic**: malaise, lethargy, fever, arthralgia, anorexia, and weight loss are common.

Signs
- **Upper airway**: septal perforation and the classic 'saddle-shaped' nasal deformity point strongly towards Wegener's granulomatosis but are late signs.
- **Respiratory and renal**: commonly little specific to find.
- **Systemic**: low-grade pyrexia, vasculitic rash.

Investigations

Determining the diagnosis and exact type of vasculitis is important as it determines therapy. Routine laboratory tests and imaging will raise suspicion; specific diagnosis is made by a combination of autoantibody pattern and biopsy.

Urine
If renal involvement, positive dipstick test for blood and protein. Red cell casts seen on microscopy indicate active glomerulonephritis.

Blood
- Routine bloods, including FBC, U&Es, clotting.
- ESR/CRP.
- Creatine kinase.
- Blood cultures.
- Autoantibodies
  - Antinuclear antibody (ANA), including anti-double-stranded DNA.
  - Antineutrophil cytoplasmic antibodies (ANCA): levels and type (c-ANCA/anti-PR3 or p-ANCA/anti-MPO).
  - Anti-glomerular basement membrane antibodies (anti-GBM).
- Other immunological tests including serum immunoglobulins and protein electrophoresis, complement levels, hepatitis B and C serology, ASO titres.

Chest radiograph
- Diffuse alveolar haemorrhage appears as bilateral patchy alveolar shadows. The differential includes infection or pulmonary oedema.
- Wegener's granulomatosis can produce a myriad of appearances (cavitation, pulmonary nodules, consolidation) and can mimic malignancy.

Arterial blood gases
- Hypoxaemia and hypocapnia result in an elevated A–a gradient due to alveolar haemorrhage.
- Elevated serum lactate can imply tissue hypoperfusion.

CT chest and sinuses

- Bony destruction of the sinuses can occur in Wegener's granulomatosis.
- Alveolar haemorrhage appears as diffuse ground glass change.
- In the acute setting CT thorax is of most use if an alternative cause of haemoptysis is considered.

Pulmonary function tests

- The textbook finding of an elevated corrected transfer factor (KCO) is good for monitoring response to therapy but is of little use acutely.

Biopsy

- Diagnosis is generally confirmed by a tissue biopsy from a site of active disease, depending on presentation (e.g. nasopharyngeal lesion, renal biopsy). Lung biopsy is performed in the absence of renal involvement. Transbronchial biopsy at bronchoscopy is rarely diagnostic and thoracoscopic or open lung biopsy is required.
- When clinical features are typical and supported by autoantibody pattern (see classification above), a biopsy is occasionally unnecessary.

Management

For the on-call physician the management of pulmonary–renal syndromes should be as follows.

- Consider the diagnosis and its differentials.
- Assess the severity, in particular the level of organ dysfunction and need for critical care support.
- Ensure all the appropriate tests have been done.
- Liaise with an appropriate specialist for ongoing care. Nephrologists, respiratory physicians, or rheumatologists commonly manage these vasculitides.
- Initiate therapy if needed. Untreated Wegener's granulomatosis, microscopic polyangiitis, and Goodpasture's disease have a poor prognosis. Early initiation of immunosuppression can be both life- and organ-saving. If the suspicion is high enough, the correct tests have been sent off, and there is organ dysfunction, immunosuppression is indicated.

Corticosteroids

- High-dose oral prednisolone up to 60 mg/day.
- High-dose IV methylprednisolone if very unwell: 500 mg for 3 days, then change to oral prednisolone as above.

Cyclophosphamide

Should be started with corticosteroids; there is no place for steroids alone.

- Oral cyclophosphamide: 2 mg/kg/day up to 150 mg.
- IV cyclophosphamide: 600 mg/m^2.

Plasmapheresis/plasma exchange
- May improve outcome in variety of autoimmune conditions including Goodpasture's disease and Wegener's granulomatosis.
- Requires the involvement of haematology, nephrology, or critical care teams.

Patients remain under long-term specialist management as immunosuppression is required long term and disease relapses can occur.

Further reading

OHRM, Chapter 41.

Griffiths M, Brett S (2003). The pulmonary physician in critical care. Illustrative case 3: pulmonary vasculitis. *Thorax*, **58**, 543–6.

Tuberculosis

① Tuberculosis

Tuberculosis (TB) remains a major worldwide health problem. The WHO estimates that a third of the world's population is currently infected with the TB bacillus, with nine million new cases and two million deaths per year. About 5–10% of those infected with TB bacilli become sick or infectious at some point in their life, and those with HIV have increased risk of developing TB.

The highest incidence of TB and the highest mortality occurs in sub-Saharan Africa. TB incidence continues to increase worldwide, particularly in Africa, where it is rising in line with the spread of HIV. Incidence has increased in the UK to more than 8000 new cases per year, with the highest rates in London and in those born outside the UK.

Pathophysiology

TB is a contagious disease caused by *Mycobacterium tuberculosis*, also known as Koch's bacillus, which is an acid-fast bacillus spread via airborne droplet nuclei. Only those with pulmonary TB are infectious. Once a person becomes infected with TB, the infection can take a number of different courses:

- The immune system may kill the bacillus.
- The bacillus may cause primary TB.
- The bacillus may become dormant and remain asymptomatic.
- The bacillus may reactivate. This can occur either after primary TB or a period of asymptomatic latency.

Clinical presentation

Pulmonary TB

Usually presents with a history of productive cough, often with haemoptysis, associated with fever, night sweats, weight loss, and anorexia.

Tuberculous lymphadenitis

Presents with enlarged lymph nodes anywhere in the body, sometimes painful, ± systemic malaise. Most common site is the unilateral cervical lymph nodes.

Skeletal TB

Usually presents with pain in the affected area (most frequently the spine but can occur anywhere), often with associated systemic upset including fever, sweats and weight loss. If occurring in the joint then usually only affects a single joint; hip and knee more than other joints.

TB meningitis

Presents with persistent headache for days to weeks ± fever. May have associated altered conscious level or focal neurology.

Other

Other sites include genitourinary, gastrointestinal, psoas abscesses, and cutaneous TB (known as lupus vulgaris when occurring on extremities). GI TB can occur at any point along the GI tract and may present with malabsorption. GU TB may present like pyelonephritis, although in men it can present as epididymitis or a scrotal mass, whilst in women it can present as pelvic inflammatory disease.

Disseminated disease

Miliary pattern may be seen on CXR.

More common in those with immunosuppression, and associated with a higher mortality.

Differential diagnosis of pulmonary TB

- Atypical mycobacterium.
- Malignancy.

Investigation

This depends in part on the site involved. Pulmonary TB should be investigated as follows.

- CXR.
- At least three early morning sputum samples for AFB and culture.
- FBC, U&E, LFTS, and CRP.
- Consider Mantoux test: intradermal injection of purified protein derivative, read at 48 hours. Size of induration is diagnostic.
  - <5 mm: negative
  - 5–14 mm: positive
  - >15 mm: strongly positive
- Bronchoscopy and lavage if sputum negative. In children, consider induced sputum or gastric washings (as AFBs in sputum are swallowed overnight and hence can be yielded from gastric washings).

Other investigations depend on the site (see Table 30.1).

All patients with suspected TB should undergo a CXR. It is recommended that all patients diagnosed with TB should have HIV serology sent. If TB is strongly suspected, treatment should be started prior to positive culture results and continued even in the presence of negative culture results.

Treatment

Quadruple therapy is recommended as first-line treatment in all cases of TB.

- Rifampicin.
- Isoniazid.
- Pyrazinamide.
- Ethambutol.

The current regime recommends all of the above drugs for 2 months, followed by rifampicin and isoniazid alone for 4 months.

The UK Medical Research Council has shown cure rates >95% with this regimen. Supplementation with pyridoxine (to prevent peripheral neuropathy with isoniazid) is only recommended in those in whom malnourishment is felt to be a concern, such as pregnancy, alcoholism, or the homeless. Treatment is for 6 months for all TB sites except meningeal TB where a minimum of 12 months is required because of penetration across the blood–brain barrier.

Treatment with more than one drug is aimed at preventing resistance and enhancing efficacy. Rifampicin and isoniazid are the two most important drugs used currently (both are bactericidal), with rifampicin being the most important in terms of reducing duration of treatment and ensuring favourable outcome. The side effects and doses of the standard drugs are shown in Table 30.2.

Multi-drug-resistant TB

Strains of TB that are resistant to a single drug are now documented in every country. Drug-resistant TB is caused by partial or inconsistent treatment, non-compliance, or prescription of incorrect drugs. Risk factors for having resistant TB include the following.

- Previous anti-TB treatment/treatment failure.
- Contact with known case of resistant TB.
- HIV infection.
- Birth in a high-incidence country.
- Living in London.
- Age 25–44.
- Male sex.

The most common form of resistant TB seen in the UK is isoniazid resistance, which is seen in up to 6% of those of African and Indian sub-continent origin, and tends to occur in small pockets around the country. The recommended regime for isoniazid-resistant TB is rifampicin, pyrazinamide, ethambutol, and streptomycin for 2 months followed by rifampicin and ethambutol for 7 months.

MDR TB is particularly dangerous. It is defined as TB resistance to at least isoniazid and rifampicin, the two most important antibiotics in the treatment of TB. MDR TB is treatable but requires longer courses of treatment (up to 2 years) which are often more toxic to patients and more expensive.

In general, five or more antibiotics are used initially and then reduced to three or four antibiotics to which the bacillus is known to be sensitive. A regime usually consists of three or four oral antibiotics, including those from the first-line regimen to which the bacillus is sensitive and second-line treatments including macrolides and quinolones, as well as an injectable antibiotic such as an aminoglycoside.

Table 30.1 Investigations for different TB sites

Site	Imaging	Biopsy	Culture
Lymph node		Node	Node or aspirate
Bone/joint	Plain X-ray CT MRI	Site of disease	Biopsy of paraspinal abscess Site or joint fluid
GI	USS CT abdomen	Omentum Bowel	Biopsy Ascites
GU	IVU USS	Site of disease	Early-morning urine Site of disease Endometrial curettings
Disseminated	HRCT thorax USS abdomen	Lung Liver Bone marrow	Bronchial wash Liver Bone marrow Blood culture
CNS	CT brain/MRI	Tuberculoma	CSF
Skin		Site of disease	Site of disease
Pericardium	Echo	Pericardium	Pericardial fluid
Cold/liver abscess	USS	Site of disease	Site of disease

Table 30.2 First-line drugs and side effects

Drug	Daily dose	Adverse effects
Rifampicin	450 mg if <50 kg 600 mg if >50 kg	Orange body secretions (avoid contact lenses), hepatitis, nausea, renal failure, thrombocytopenia, drug interactions (CyP450 pathway)
Isoniazid	5–10 mg/kg (max 300 mg)	Hepatitis, peripheral neuropathy, drug-induced lupus
Pyrazinamide	1.5 g if <50 kg 2 g if >50 kg	Rash, nausea, hyperuricaemia, arthropathy
Ethambutol	15 mg/kg	Optic neuritis

HIV and TB

HIV infection is the strongest risk factor for developing TB. Mechanisms include the following:

- reactivation of latent TB.
- rapidly progressive primary infection.
- reinfection.

Manifestation of TB in early HIV will mimic presentation in uninfected individuals, whilst in later HIV infection it is more likely to have an atypical pulmonary presentation or be extrathoracic.

TB is the leading cause of death amongst those infected with HIV, accounting for approximately 13% of AIDS deaths worldwide. Anti-tuberculous treatment is equally effective in those who are HIV positive as in those who are HIV negative, although the treatment raises some key issues:

- increased malabsorption.
- drug–drug interaction.
- increased non-compliance.
- increased rate of relapse.
- IRIS.

It is recommended that, in those with a concurrent diagnosis of TB, the start of highly active anti-retroviral treatment (HAART) is delayed until the TB has been partially or even fully treated. This is to avoid immune reconstitution inflammatory syndrome (IRIS). Initiation of HAART has been shown to produce a sustained rise in the CD4 count, leading to a restoration of immunity to the mycobacterial antigen, which in turn causes a clinical and radiological deterioration in those with TB. The median onset of IRIS in patients with TB is 12 days after the initiation of HAART. It is usually mild and self-limiting but may respond to corticosteroids if required. Currently guidelines in general recommend delaying HAART for 2 months after starting anti-tuberculous drugs. However, there is no absolute consensus on this (☐ Chapter 33).

Protease inhibitors and non-nucleoside reverse transcriptase inhibitors are metabolized via the cytochrome p-450 pathway. Therefore they interfere with the metabolism of rifampicin and should be avoided.

TB in pregnancy

TB presents in the same way as in non-pregnant individuals, although diagnosis may be delayed because of hesitation to do a CXR in early pregnancy. Malaise may be mistaken for pregnancy symptoms in the first trimester. The Mantoux test can be performed in pregnancy and the result is not altered. The outcome of TB is the same as in non-pregnant individuals, though late diagnosis increases the risk of IUGR, pre-eclampsia, stillbirth, and obstetric mortality.

Treatment

The standard 6 month regimen of rifampicin, isoniazid, pyrazinamide, and ethambutol is recommended. There are limited data on the teratogenicity of pyrazinamide, although the other three drugs are not teratogenic. Second-line treatments should be used with caution as they may be toxic. The risk of congenital infection or infection at delivery is extremely rare. Babies born to a smear-positive (sputum) mother (still in the first 2 weeks of treatment) should have prophylactic isoniazid with a skin test at 6 weeks. Breast feeding is also safe with the usual anti-tuberculous drugs.

① Patient presenting with a known diagnosis of tuberculosis

Infection risk

Those with smear-positive TB, i.e. those who have sputum positive for AFB on microscopy, are infectious until completion of the first 2 weeks of anti-tuberculous chemotherapy. All other patients with TB are non-infectious.

Drug side effects

The most frequent side effects of the four commonly used anti-tuberculous drugs are shown in Table 30.2.

If visual acuity is affected, ethambutol should be stopped immediately and replaced, if necessary, by a second-line drug such as streptomycin, a macrolide, or a quinolone. Advice should be sought from the treating chest physician.

If liver toxicity occurs, it is often difficult to identify the causative drug. Liver toxicity is defined as

> AST/ALT rise 5× normal or bilirubin rise

In these cases, rifampicin, isoniazid, and pyrazinamide need to be stopped. Ethambutol can be continued, and if the patient is unwell or still smear-positive then consider use of second-line therapy (such as streptomycin) until oral drugs can be reinstituted.

Once liver function tests have returned to baseline, the drugs can be reintroduced one at a time as follows.

- Isoniazid at 50 mg/day. Sequential increase to 300 mg/day over 3–4 days if no adverse effects.
- Rifampicin at 75 mg/day. Increase slowly to 300 mg/day over same time frame if no adverse effects; then increase to maximum dose.
- Pyrazinamide at 250 mg/day; then increase to 1 g/day over 2–3 days and then to the maximum dose if no adverse effects.

Measure LFT and review clinical state on a daily basis.

If no further reaction, continue with full chemotherapy as initiated.

If there is a further reaction to one of the drugs, exclude and change to an alternative regime. If pyrazinamide is not tolerated, an alternative regime of rifampicin and isoniazid for 9 months with ethambutol for the first 2 months can be used.

Other effects of anti-tuberculous drugs

Table 30.3 Interactions with other drugs

Drug	Increases level	Decreases level
Rifampicin		OCP
		Warfarin
		Phenytoin
		Carbamazepine
		Barbiturates
		Sulphonylureas
		Corticosteroids
		Cyclosporin
Isoniazid	Phenytoin	
	Carbamazepine	
	Warfarin	

Worsening clinical condition or CXR changes
Consider the following.
- In some patients, there is an initial worsening of condition (e.g. increased size of lymph nodes or worsening of CXR changes) because of a degree of immune reconstitution. Consider treatment with oral steroids.
- Non-compliance.
- In HIV patients started on HAART, consider immune reconstitution.
- Concomitant community- or hospital-acquired infection.
- Alternative diagnosis (particularly with mediastinal lymphadenopathy; consider lymphoma or sarcoidosis).

Part 4

Chronic respiratory conditions

Chronic respiratory conditions

Bronchiectasis

① Bronchiecstasis

Bronchiectasis is a descriptive term given to the condition of chronic dilation of one or more airways, resulting in poor mucus clearance and hence recurrent or chronic bacterial infection. Only 40% of cases have an identifiable cause. (For more information, see OHRM, Chapter 29).

Common treatment points

- Patients tend to be infected by *Haemophilus influenzae* early in their course, then *Staphylococcus aureus*, *Moraxella catarrhalis*, and finally *Pseudomonas aeruginosa*.
- Management includes daily chest physiotherapy, nutritional support, and sometimes prophylactic antibiotics.
- Patients chronically colonized with *Pseudomonas aeruginosa* may use regular aerosol anti-pseudomonas antibiotics to reduce the bacterial load.
- If evidence of an asthmatic component to disease, inhaled steroids are sometimes used.
- Patients may have had a previous lobectomy or pneumonectomy, as surgery used to be a common form of treatment for this condition.

Pulmonary exacerbation

- Symptoms: ↑cough, ↑dyspnoea, change in sputum (volume, colour, thickness), pleuritic pain, lethargy.
- Signs: airway secretions, wheeze, crackles, rubs, ↓ FEV_1, CXR changes.
- Investigations: FBC, U&Es, CRP, sputum for MC&S, exclude pneumothorax, check total IgE and aspergillus RAST (for ABPA, see below), check ABG if SaO_2 <93% or if there is ventilatory insufficiency.
- Treatment: the aim is to see an improvement in symptoms, sputum, FEV_1, and CRP.
  - The choice of antibiotic is influenced by the colonizing organism. The patient may have a self-management plan with a course of antibiotics ready to start at home.
  - For mild exacerbations, high-dose oral antibiotics should be given for 10–14 days. If colonizing organism not known, treat with amoxicillin (0.5–1 g tds) until sputum microbiology available.
  - For severe exacerbations, IV antibiotics chosen according to sputum microbiology should be given for 10–14 days. Consider oxygen or non-invasive ventilation.
  - If colonized with P. aeruginosa, use ciprofloxacin 750 mg bd for mild exacerbations. If this treatment fails or the exacerbation is moderate/severe, then IV antibiotics should be administered.
  - Anti-pseudomonal IV antibiotics should include a β-lactam (e.g. ceftazidime 1–2 g tds, meropenem 1–2 g tds, or piperacillin/tazobactam (Tazocin®) 4.5–6.75 g tds) combined with an aminoglycoside (e.g. gentamicin or tobramycin) given once daily according to hospital protocol (usually 5–7 mg/kg at 10 p.m. followed by levels at 8 a.m. which are then cross-referenced on a dosing table).

- Airway clearance, either individual active clearance techniques or with assistance from physiotherapist. Urgent physiotherapist input not needed out of hours unless the patient is very unwell.
- Consider bronchodilators prior to physiotherapy to treat wheeze and aid expectoration.

Mucus plugging of the airway

- Symptoms: as for pulmonary exacerbation. Sputum may be thick and difficult to expectorate or contain plugs.
- Signs: may lead to collapse or consolidation distal to the plug on examination or CXR.
- Investigations: as for pulmonary exacerbations, with IgE and aspergillus RAST particularly important.
- Treatment
  - Nebulized bronchodilators.
  - Regular chest physiotherapy (urgently if the patient is significantly unwell).
  - IV antibiotic treatment.
  - If acute deterioration, urgent bronchoscopy may be required.
  - Consider DNase, particularly in CF.

Allergic bronchopulmonary aspergillosis (ABPA)

Definition

A heightened immune reaction against inhaled Aspergillus. After inhalation of spores of *Aspergillus fumigatus*, the fungus proliferates in the bronchial tree provoking an immune hypersensitivity reaction. This leads to eosinophilic plugs infiltrated by Aspergillus hyphae causing distal lobar or segmental collapse and thickened sputum, . May occur in bronchiectasis and is also a cause of bronchiectasis.

Diagnosis

Dyspnoea, wheeze, increased airflow obstruction on spirometry, thick sputum with dark plugs, sputum/blood eosinophilia, flitting infiltrates or collapse on CXR, raised total IgE (>1000 mg/ml), positive precipitating antibodies to Aspergillus (>90%), positive skin-prick test against Aspergillus or RAST test (100%). Presence of fungal hyphae in the sputum helps to confirm the diagnosis.

Treatment

- Oral steroids (e.g. 40 mg prednisolone) for 2 weeks, then tapered over 3 months.
- Regular chest physiotherapy (urgently if the patient is significantly unwell).
- Bronchodilators.
- Consider itraconazole 200 mg bd (for the first 16 weeks of treatment).

For further information see OHRM, Chapter 23.

Pneumothorax 📖 Chapter 26.

Haemoptysis 📖 Chapter 6.

Cystic fibrosis

⊙ Introduction

Cystic fibrosis (CF) is an inherited disease which is now as common in adults as in children. Patients born now have a predicted life expectancy of >40 years. Milder forms may be diagnosed later in life.

Mutations of the CFTR gene (coding for a chloride channel) cause thickened secretions in the lumen of the viscera. The main result is bronchiectasis with chronic airway infection, but the sinuses, pancreas, hepatobiliary system, kidneys, and reproductive tracts are also affected.

CF patients are usually managed by a multidisciplinary team at a regional CF centre and contact should be made with them (contact details available from www.cftrust.org.uk) as early as possible. Information from the patient and their notes will aid diagnosis and treatment.

Common treatment points

Respiratory

Patients should be nursed in a side-room if possible, to avoid cross-infection with different strains of *Pseudomonas aeruginosa* and other Gram-negative bacteria, particularly *Burkholderia cepacia*.

- 80% of adults are chronically colonized with *P.aeruginosa*.
- Oral antibiotics are often used to suppress *Staphylococcus aureus* or MRSA (e.g. two of rifampicin, trimethoprim, fusidic acid, and doxycycline).
- Azithromycin 250–500 mg od is often used for its anti-inflammatory properties in chronic mucoid Pseudomonas colonization.
- Prednisolone ± itraconazole 200 mg bd may be used against ABPA.
- Nebulized DNase (Pulmozyme®) or hypertonic saline is often used daily to reduce sputum viscosity before chest physiotherapy. DNase denatures nebulized antibiotics and should not be used within 1 hour of their administration.
- Aerosol anti-pseudomonas antibiotics are used to reduce *P.aeruginosa* burden in the lungs: Colomycin® (colistin) 1–2 MU bd, aminoglycosides 80–160 mg bd, Tobi® 300 mg bd in alternate months (preservative-free tobramycin preparation). These are usually given after chest physiotherapy.
- Patients needing frequent IV antibiotics may have an implanted vascular access device (a central line terminating in a subcutaneous drum-shaped device) which is accessed by specially designed needles. May become blocked or, rarely, infected.

Abdominal

- Dietary supplements (including high-calorie drinks, nasogastric or PEG tube feeding) are often needed to maintain BMI >19.
- Vitamin supplements are taken by most patients, and bisphosphonates by some, because of malabsorption and a high risk of osteoporosis.

- Proton pump inhibitors are often taken to reduce oesophageal reflux.
- Creon or pancrease tablets are taken with meals and snacks to replace deficient pancreatic enzymes.
- N-acetylcysteine 400 mg sachets (fluimucil) are sometimes taken tds–qds as prophylaxis against DIOS (see below).
- Ursodeoxycholic acid may be taken to slow the rate of progression of CF-related liver disease.
- Slow-sodium 'salt tablets' are used (from four per day in the UK to 16 per day when in hot climates) because of excess salt loss in sweat.
- Insulin and oral hypoglycaemic agents are used for CF-related diabetes.

① Pulmonary exacerbations

Presentation

A pulmonary exacerbation is defined as the presence of at least three of the following 11 new findings or changes in clinical status when compared with the most recent baseline visit.
- Increased cough.
- Increased sputum production and/or a change in appearance of expectorated sputum.
- Fever (>37.9°C for at least 4 hours in a 24 hour period) on more than one occasion in the previous week.
- Weight loss >1 kg or 5% of body weight associated with anorexia and decreased dietary intake or growth failure in an infant or child.
- School or work absenteeism (due to illness) in the previous week.
- Increased respiratory rate and/or work of breathing.
- New findings on chest examination (e.g. crackles and wheezes).
- Decreased exercise tolerance.
- Decrease in FEV_1 (of more than 10% from previous baseline study).
- Decrease in oxygen saturation (of more than 10% from previous baseline value).
- New findings on CXR.

Investigations

- Sputum for MC&S.
- CXR to exclude pneumothorax.
- Check blood sugars (before and after meals).
- Check total IgE and Aspergillus RAST (for ABPA, 📖 Chapter 31), check U&Es.
- Check ABG if SaO_2 <93% or if ventilatory insufficiency suspected.

Treatment

See Table 32.1 for antibiotic choice.
- Chest physiotherapy at least daily (not needed out of hours unless the patient is very unwell).
- Minor exacerbations may be treated with oral antibiotics. If more than two of the 11 symptoms or signs of exacerbation are present (or otherwise clinically indicated) IV antibiotics are indicated, and should be given via a long line or a Venflon with a bacterial filter. Antibiotic

choice depends on usual sputum microbiology and which antibiotics usually work (ask the patient). *In vitro* sensitivities are often unhelpful for *P.aeruginosa* and *B.cepacia* complex. If no known chronic colonizing bacteria, aim to treat *Haemophilus influenzae,* which is a common cause of exacerbation. Tobramycin or gentamicin can be dosed once daily using your local protocol. Dosing three times daily can be done as follows: if weight <50 kg start with 80 mg tds, otherwise start with 100 mg tds; check levels on third to fifth dose (aiming pre-dose <2 mg/L and 1 hour post-dose 8–12 mg/L). Nebulized antibiotics are often stopped if the same antibiotic is given IV, but this is not crucial.

- If worsening despite antibiotics, check sputum results and antibiotic sensitivities, repeat sputum, and rule out haemoptysis, pneumothorax, ABPA, mucus plugging, and poor glycaemic control.
- If necessary, other measures may be added, similar to COPD treatment: oxygen (beware CO_2 retention), nebulized bronchodilators, IV aminophylline, oral or IV steroids (only if absolutely necessary), or non-invasive ventilation.

Table 32.1 Antibiotic choice in infective exacerbations of CF

Bacterium	Oral antibiotics	IV antibiotics
H.influenzae	One of:	One of:
	Amoxicillin 0.5–1 g tds	Amoxicillin 0.5–1 g tds
	Co-amoxiclav	Co-amoxiclav
	Tetracycline	Third-generation cephalosporin
	Macrolide	
S.aureus	One of:	One of:
	Flucloxacillin 0.25–0.5 g qds (± fucidic acid)	Flucloxacillin 0.25–2 g qds
	Macrolide	Macrolide
	Tetracycline	Second-generation cephalosporin
	Clindamycin	
P.aeruginosa	Ciprofloxacin 750 mg bd	One of:
		Ceftazidime 2 g tds
		Aztreonam 2 g tds
		Meropenem 1 g tds
		Piperacillin/tazobactam (Tazocin®) 4.5–6.75 g tds
		PLUS one of:
		Tobramycin
		Gentamicin
		Colistin (2 MU tds)
B.cepacia complex	One of:	As for P.aeruginosa but use two β-lactams
	Doxycycline/minocycline	PLUS an aminoglycoside
	Macrolide	Do not use colistin
	Co-trimoxazole	
	Chloramphenicol	

Mucus plugging of the airways, ABPA

Should be treated as for bronchiectasis (📖 Chapter 33).

Haemoptysis and pneumothorax

📖 Chapters 6 and 26.

① Biochemical abnormalities

- Salt loss may cause dehydration and lethargy during hot weather. Replace salt and water orally or IV (0.9% saline) depending on severity.
- Hypomagnesaemia may cause lethargy. Replace with an infusion especially if also on an aminoglycoside (e.g. 20 mmol $MgSO_4$ in 500 ml saline over 6 hours). Oral magnesium glycerophosphate two tablets tds may help, but is very poorly absorbed.

① Distal intestinal obstruction syndrome (DIOS)

- Thickened secretions in the intestines may cause subacute partial obstruction or even acute obstruction.
- Often triggered by dehydration, poor glycaemic control, change in diet, or change in pancreatic enzyme use.
- If mild, rehydrate and add fibre and lactulose.
- If severe, treat with gastrografin 100 ml with 400 ml water od for 1–5 days.
- If no better use Klean-Prep via nasogastric tube.

Further information

OHRM, Chapter 30.

Notes on various emergencies are available online at: http://www.cftrust.org.uk/aboutcf/publications/

HIV and the lung

① Introduction

Human immunodeficiency virus (HIV) infection can cause a number of conditions within the lung depending on the degree of immunosuppression. It is responsible for a number of problems within the lung. Many of these conditions are also seen in other immunosuppressed patients (📖 Chapter 13), although the prognosis can be very different.

In patients with a low CD4 count the differential diagnosis of dyspnoea and CXR abnormalities is wide, including PCP, Mycobacteria (TB and non-TB), Aspergillus, Lymphoma, Kaposi's sarcoma, LIP, CMV, Cryptococcus, Histoplasmosis, Candida, Toxoplasmosis, viruses, Nocardia, and Actinomyces.

Additionally HIV is a risk factor for developing lymphoma (typically non-Hodgkin's) and primary lung cancer.

① Tuberculosis

There is an increased risk of developing both tuberculous and non-tuberculous mycobacterial infection with HIV. This is a specialist area and involvement of an HIV specialist is advised.

The current recommendations for TB and HIV management from NICE are those of the British HIV Association.

- For fully sensitive TB not involving the CNS:
  - Standard anti-tuberculous treatment (📖 Chapter 30).
  - If sputum remains smear-positive at 2 months the continuation phase should be extended to 7 months.
- For fully sensitive TB involving the CNS:
  - Standard initial phase followed by 10 months continuation phase.
- For multidrug-resistant TB:
  - 2 years of treatment may be required and the patient should be referred to a specialist centre.

Rifampicin should not be used in combination with non-nucleoside reverse transcription inhibitors and protease inhibitors as they interact.

The question of when to start highly active anti-retroviral therapy (HAART) in someone who has been diagnosed with both TB and HIV has not been clearly defined. Drug interactions, toxicity, and side effects with both HAART and anti-tuberculous medication make co-administration a potential problem. The current recommendations are based on the CD4 count at the time of initiation of anti-TB therapy.

- CD4 count >200 cells/μL: delay HAART until 6 months of TB therapy completed.
- CD4 count 100–200 cells/μL: start HAART after 2 months initial therapy completed.
- CD4 count <100 cells/μL: start HAART as soon as possible based on physician assessment (some delay for 2 months).

Immune reconstitution inflammatory syndrome can occur when HAART is initiated (see tuberculosis chapter).

① Pneumocystis pneumonia (PCP)

Pneumocystis jiroveci (previously called *Pneumocystis carinii*) is a fungal organism. Immunocompromised individuals are at risk of developing pneumocystis pneumonia. The incidence has fallen in solid organ transplant patients and HIV patients with use of prophylaxis. Also HAART has helped to reduce the frequency of PCP. It is uncommon in HIV patients with a CD4 count >200 cells/μL.

Signs and symptoms

- Persistent non-productive cough.
- Dyspnoea.
- Fevers.
- Chest discomfort.
- Hypoxia.
- Tachypnoea.
- Tachycardia.
- Chest auscultation: typically normal though inspiratory crackles/ wheeze may be present.

PCP can affect other organs resulting in hepatomegaly, bone marrow necrosis, retinal 'cotton-wool spots', skin lesions, thyroid masses, or lymphadenopathy.

Investigations

Similar to investigations for bacterial pneumonia.

- CXR: appearance can be very variable. Classically shows diffuse bilateral infiltrates but it may show focal infiltrates, thin-walled cysts, or pneumothorax, or simply appear normal.
- ABG as PaO_2 is used to assess severity:
  - mild (PaO_2 >11 kPa).
  - moderate (PaO_2 8–11 kPa).
  - Severe (PaO_2 <8 kPa).

If resting oxygen saturations are normal and the diagnosis is suspected, measure SaO_2 on exertion to look for desaturation.

- CD4 count.
- High LDH levels are common.
- Sputum for Gram stain and culture has a low yield in PCP, but should also be sent for mycobacteria.
- Serology for atypical pathogens and CMV should also be considered.
- Induced sputum has a higher yield but requires trained staff (and carries the risk of spreading other infectious agents, e.g. TB).
- Bronchoscopy and lavage to obtain samples for PCP staining or immunofluorescence.
- CT thorax can show patchy ground glass opacification with interlobular septal thickening.
- Open-lung biopsy will give tissue for histology and is the most reliable test for PCP. However, it is also very invasive.

Treatment

Consider starting empirically if high level of suspicion, as there can be delays in obtaining a microbiological diagnosis. Treatment should be continued for 21 days (14 days treatment may be sufficient for non-HIV PCP).

- Co-trimoxazole orally or IV, 120 mg/kg daily in two to four divided doses for all categories of severity.
- Prednisolone 50–80 mg daily should be given in moderate or severe cases. Wean the dose after 5 days and stop prior to finishing the co-trimoxazole course.

Alternative treatment if allergic/intolerant to co-trimoxazole.

- Mild to moderate disease:
  - atovaquone 750 mg bd.
  - dapsone (100 mg od) with trimethoprim (5 mg/kg every 6–8 hours).
  - clindamycin (600 mg tds) with primaquine (30 mg od).
  - nebulized pentamidine isetionate (for mild disease only) 600 mg od.
- Severe disease:
  - pentamidine isethionate IV 4 mg/kg daily (for severe disease or if there is failure to respond to co-trimoxazole).

Prognosis

Depending on severity at presentation mortality is between 10% and 50%.

Prophylaxis

HIV patients with a CD4 count <200 cells/μL should receive prophylaxis against PCP. It can be discontinued in HIV patients on HAART once their CD4 count is >200 cells/μL. For other immunosuppressed patients, prophylaxis should be considered. In solid organ transplants the optimum duration of prophylaxis is not clearly defined.

- Co-trimoxazole 960 mg daily (or three times a week) is recommended. This also provides protection against cerebral toxoplasmosis.

Alternative prophylaxis for patients unable to take co-trimoxazole.

- Dapsone 100 mg od.
- Atovaquone 750 mg bd.
- Pentamidine isethionate nebulized 300 mg every 4 weeks or 150 mg every 2 weeks (this gives pulmonary but not systemic protection against PCP).

⑦ Lymphocytic interstitial pneumonia

Lymphocytic interstitial pneumonia (LIP) is associated with all forms of immunosuppression, including HIV. It is more common in children than adults. It is caused by lymphocyte and plasma cell infiltration into the interstitium.

Symptoms are non-specific and include cough and dyspnoea. CXR appearances are bilateral infiltrates (often basal). Bronchoscopy and transbronchial biopsy can be diagnostic, although surgical lung biopsy may be necessary. Treatment is with steroids.

⑦ Kaposi's sarcoma

This is a vascular tumour associated with human herpes virus 8 co-infection. It is commonly found on the skin but can also affect the lung. Kaposi's lesions are uncommon with a CD4 count >50 cells/μL. Symptoms are cough, dyspnoea, chest pain, and haemoptysis. Kaposi's sarcoma can cause mediastinal lymphadenopathy, focal infiltrates, and nodularity on CXR. Lesions can be seen on bronchoscopy, although biopsies should be performed with caution because of their vascularity.

Treatment is with HAART, radiotherapy to localized symptomatic disease, and/or chemotherapy.

2) Lymphocytic interstitial pneumonia

3) Kaposi's sarcoma

Interstitial lung disease

Introduction

The classification of interstitial lung disease (ILD) has been refined significantly over recent years and is rather confusing to the uninitiated! Most ILDs are rare and unlikely to present as an emergency. Cryptogenic fibrosing alveolitis (CFA), also known as idiopathic pulmonary fibrosis (IPF), is probably the most frequent ILD encountered in routine respiratory practice. The pathology underlying this is termed 'usual interstitial pneumonia' (UIP) and it is one of the so-called 'idiopathic interstitial pneumonias' (IIPs). These three terms (IPF, CFA, UIP) are often used interchangeably in the same patient's notes which can easily cause further confusion! Description of the pathological distinction between specific disease entities is beyond the scope of this chapter (see OHRM, Chapter 35).

① Known idiopathic pulmonary fibrosis

IPF is a slowly progressive condition with a median survival of around 3 years. It is often difficult to predict the likely disease course at diagnosis, with some patients running a much more benign course than others. In some cases steroids and immunosuppressives can promote disease stability and so may be used long term in this condition.

The most frequent scenario causing a diagnostic problem is of the patient with IPF presenting with increased breathlessness with no specific diagnostic pointers. Causes to consider are the following.

- Natural disease progression: suggested by more insidious than acute progression of symptoms.
- Infection: associated fever, cough, sputum.
- Pulmonary thromboembolism (PTE): acute deterioration in SOB.
- Pneumothorax: treat as secondary pneumothorax.
- Accelerated disease phase/IPF 'exacerbation'.

Assessment

- CXR: progressive reticular change suggests disease progression, but CXR is frequently insensitive in its detection. May be difficult to determine definite consolidation in a patient with significant fibrosis. Look carefully for small pneumothoraces.
- Blood tests: worth checking inflammatory markers/white cell count. Significant elevation suggests infection. A negative D-dimer is helpful in the exclusion of PTE.
- CTPA: often needed if no clear diagnosis from initial assessment. Will clarify PTE/consolidation. V/Q scanning is not helpful.

Management

Manage PTE/infection as standard, although have a lower threshold for broad-spectrum/severe pneumonia antimicrobial cover. Treat pneumothorax as per secondary pneumothorax protocol (□ Page 170).

If infection is present, stop immunosuppressives. Steroids should be continued and if the patient has been on them long term, consider transient increase in dose to cover the period of infection.

IPF exacerbation

If infection, PTE, and other causes of breathlessness are confidently excluded, consideration must be given to accelerated disease/IPF 'exacerbation'. This increasingly recognized phenomenon is often characterized by preceding fever/influenza-like illness, respiratory failure, and dramatic progression of parenchymal abnormalities (ground glass opacification on CT). Pathologically these patients have findings of diffuse alveolar damage. High-dose steroids (possibly with IV methylprednisolone) may be helpful, although this disease complication is associated with a poor prognosis.

① **Other idiopathic interstitial lung diseases**

The majority of interstitial lung diseases, including non-specific interstitial pneumonia (NSIP), respiratory bronchiolitis-associated interstitial lung disease (RBILD), and lymphocytic interstitial pneumonitis (LIP), are generally seen and managed in outpatient chest clinics. Those conditions that are more likely to present acutely are briefly discussed below.

While quite different radiologically and pathologically, in general all these conditions are associated with a better prognosis than IPF/UIP and have a more favourable response to anti-inflammatory and/or immunosuppressive treatment. A similar approach to that described above should be adopted if these conditions present with respiratory symptoms as an emergency.

As a general rule, it is best not to increase or initiate steroids in such patients unless respiratory failure is so significant that this decision is being pressed. Specialist advice should be sought.

Cryptogenic organizing pneumonia

- Presents with influenza-like illness, with cough, fever, malaise, and weight loss.
- <2 months of symptoms in 75% of cases.
- ESR and CRP raised.
- Multifocal and/or flitting consolidation on CXR.
- 50% of cases are truly 'cryptogenic'. The remainder may be triggered by a variety of conditions, e.g. infection, connective tissue disorder, drug reaction, post bone marrow or lung transplant, inflammatory bowel disease.
- Diagnosis suggested by HRCT and usually confirmed on transbronchial biopsy.
- Good response to steroids in 80% of cases.

Acute interstitial pneumonia
- Previously known as Hamman–Rich syndrome.
- Presents with initial influenza-like illness, with cough, fever, malaise, and weight loss followed by rapidly progressive dyspnoea.
- <3 weeks of symptoms in most cases. Usually hypoxic at presentation.
- Extensive alveolar shadowing on CXR; costophrenic angles often spared.
- Diagnosed with HRCT, transbronchial biopsy, or lung biopsy.
- Specialist management (may need BAL to exclude infection).
- Response to steroids often disappointing. Mortality >50%.

① Drug-induced interstitial lung disease

A huge spectrum of specific lung pathologies is encompassed in the above term. The best source of specific information about suspected drug-induced lung injury is www.pneumotox.com.

Difficulties arise in that frequently different potential manifestations may occur from the same drug (e.g. amiodarone can cause subacute cellular pneumonitis, organizing pneumonia, and pulmonary fibrosis, to name but three effects), and the drug in question may have been discontinued some time before the onset of symptoms (examples of later presentations include nitrosoureas, radiotherapy, and amiodarone). However, the drug is usually still being taken at the time of presentation and has been taken for at least weeks and up to years.

Drugs most commonly causing ILD include the following.
- Amiodarone.
- Methotrexate.
- Cyclophosphamide.
- Gold.
- Penicillamine.
- Sulfasalazine.
- Nitrofurantoin.
- Cocaine.

There may be an associated peripheral blood eosinophilia.

Initial investigation and management is as for any other presentation of dyspnoea (📖 Chapter 2).

① Hypersensitivity pneumonitis (HP)

Previously termed extrinsic allergic alveolitis (EAA), HP can present acutely within 4–8 hours of exposure to the relevant antigen (e.g. mouldy hay) (see OHRM, p458).

Clinical features

Characteristically dyspnoea, dry cough, and systemic upset (e.g. fever, arthralgia, myalgia, headache) with crackles (sometimes squeaks) on auscultation. Wheeze is absent.

Investigation and diagnosis

CXR may be normal (especially if significant time has elapsed from antigen exposure), although characteristically shows diffuse small (1–3 mm) nodules or infiltrates, often sparing the apices.

Routine bloods may show elevated inflammatory markers or neutrophilia. ABG may reveal hypoxaemia.

The most helpful clue to the diagnosis is a history of recurrent episodes of symptoms that resolve following cessation of antigen exposure with the above clinical findings.

The majority of cases will not require admission or specific treatment.

Where the clinical history is compatible with the diagnosis, and in the absence of significant systemic upset or significant hypoxia:

• Counsel the patient about avoiding further antigen exposure.
• Send off blood for serum precipitin analysis.
• Arrange chest clinic follow up (to ensure resolution of infiltrates or further investigation if needed).

Arrange HRCT (characteristically shows patchy ground glass change and poorly defined nodules) and respiratory review. Corticosteroids may be needed. Atypical presentations will require further investigation (bronchoscopy with lavage and transbronchial lung biopsy or occasionally surgical lung biopsy) to exclude alternative pathology.

Sarcoidosis

⑦ Sarcoidosis

Sarcoidosis is a multisystem inflammatory disorder of unknown cause. It is a relatively rare condition (UK incidence 5–10 in 100 000) and so it is unusual for it to present in the acute medical setting.

Acute sarcoid, previously undiagnosed, may present as Löfgren's syndrome, a combination of erythema nodosum, bilateral hilar lymphadenopathy on the CXR, fever, and arthralgia. This requires no specific treatment (other than simple analgesics or NSAIDs for arthralgia/pain from erythema nodosum) and has an excellent prognosis; the majority will resolve completely within 1–2 years.

In the above situation it is worth checking baseline renal function, calcium, and ACE level (which may be raised in sarcoid, although elevated levels are not diagnostic) and referring for outpatient HRCT/PFT and chest clinic follow up to clarify degree of lymphadenopathy and lack of parenchymal involvement. In this situation biopsy of lymph nodes by mediastinoscopy (to exclude lymphoma/TB) is usually not needed unless there is anything atypical about the situation.

Known diagnosis of sarcoid

Respiratory presentation

Causes of increased shortness of breath, on a background of sarcoid, are most commonly due to the following.

Flare of sarcoid

Comparison of CXR with earlier films is important. Both sarcoid and infection can cause an increase in shadowing on the CXR and discrimination between the two can be difficult, although dense consolidation (especially lobar) is unlikely to be sarcoid. Discuss with chest team about need for starting/increasing existing dose of steroid and arranging appropriate outpatient investigation/review. In treating active disease standard treatment would be prednisolone 40 mg od for 4 weeks before tapering to a maintenance dose, ideally under review of a respiratory physician.

Infection

Treat as community-acquired infection. If the patient is on maintenance steroids, consider a transient increase in dose whilst unwell.

Pneumothorax

Occurs in cases of sarcoid with pulmonary fibrosis: treat as secondary pneumothorax.

Non-respiratory presentation

- Hypercalcaemia.
- Skin: erythema nodosum (symptomatic treatment and NSAIDs), lupus pernio, and cutaneous sarcoid.
- Cardiac sarcoidosis: most commonly presents with conduction defects. Therefore perform ECG on all sarcoid patients.
- Neurosarcoidosis: can present with any neurological symptom. Most common presentation is lower motor neuron facial palsy.
- Ocular sarcoidosis (sight-threatening): usually anterior uveitis. However episcleritis, scleritis, conjunctivitis, glaucoma, and retinal involvement can occur. Require slit-lamp examination. Refer to ophthalmology.
- Renal sarcoidosis: rarely presents with acute renal failure.

Bear in mind that other specialities may well need to be involved in care of patients with extra-pulmonary sarcoidosis. Extra-pulmonary sarcoid is often an indication for high-dose immunosuppressive treatment, particularly the following.

- Cardiac sarcoidosis.
- Neurosarcoidosis.
- Hypercalcaemia.
- Lupus pernio.
- Sight-threatening ocular sarcoidosis.
- Hepatic, splenic, or renal sarcoidosis.

Known diagnosis of lung cancer

① Introduction

Lung cancer is the most common cause of cancer death in the UK and therefore is likely to present to the acute physician at some time. This chapter deals briefly with lung cancer itself; for more detailed information see OHRM, Chapter 18. Patients with a known diagnosis of lung cancer may present acutely with symptoms due to the primary problem of the lung cancer itself (which may or may not be with primarily respiratory symptoms), complications of treatment, or a respiratory presentation due to coexisting respiratory disease.

Non-small-cell lung cancer (NSCLC)

Patients undergoing lung resection for stage I NSCLC (primary tumour <3 cm diameter, no nodal or distant disease) have a 5 year survival of 60–70%. Five year survival falls as disease stage progresses, with stage IV NSCLC (any distant disease) having a 5 year survival of <5%. Radical radiotherapy (for patients with resectable tumours but not fit for an operation) can achieve 5-year survival in up to 19% of patients. Chemotherapy for NSCLC has a small (but statistically significant) impact on survival, with median survival improved by 6–7 weeks.

Small-cell lung cancer (SCLC)

Untreated SCLC has a median survival of 6 weeks. If at presentation disease is limited stage (limited to one hemithorax) and patients show response to chemotherapy and then receive consolidation chest radiotherapy and prophylactic cranial irradiation, median survival is in the region of 14–20 months.

① Respiratory symptoms related to lung cancer

Clearly, all cardinal symptoms of respiratory disease (dyspnoea, cough, sputum, wheeze, haemoptysis, chest pain) can be present in patients with underlying lung cancer, but the most common reason for presenting as an emergency is increased dyspnoea. The reasons for presentation can be grouped into the following categories:

- Disease progression: pleural effusion, large airway obstruction, lobar collapse, SVCO, lymphangitis, pericardial effusion, diaphragmatic paralysis, chest wall infiltration.
- Complications of disease or its progression: pulmonary embolism, pneumonia (often occurring distal to the site of airway obstruction by tumour), pneumothorax, anaemia.
- Coexisting respiratory pathology: COPD, asthma, pulmonary fibrosis.

One needs to keep an open mind as the presenting respiratory diagnosis may be *unrelated* to the underlying lung cancer (e.g. RLL pneumonia in a patient with localized tumour in the LUL).

✪ Primarily non-respiratory symptoms related to lung cancer

Lung cancer most commonly metastasises to liver, bone, brain, and adrenals and may present with symptoms or signs related to this.

Remember the paraneoplastic syndromes.

The following is a brief non-exhaustive list of common presentations.

- Confusion.
  - Brain metastases.
  - SIADH:
    — hyponatraemia <125 mmol/L.
    — low plasma osmolality <260 mmol/kg.
    — concentrated urine (with sodium >20 mmol/L).
  - Hypercalcaemia.
- Bone pain/pathological fracture: bony metastases.
- Leg weakness/back pain: spinal metastases. Neurological symptoms occur with spinal cord compression.
- Electrolyte abnormalities.
  - Hyponatraemia (SIADH).
  - Hypokalaemia (ectopic ACTH).
  - Hypercalcaemia (ectopic rPTH or bony metastases).
- Miscellaneous.
  - Abdominal discomfort/swelling (liver metastases, ascites; consider constipation secondary to hypercalcaemia or opiate analgesics)
  - DVT.

✪ Attendance as a complication of therapy

Patients undergoing chemotherapy for both small-cell and non-small-cell lung cancer may present with complications of this treatment, particularly neutropaenic sepsis (treat as per hospital guidelines).

Following lung resection, risks include empyema, wound infection, and pulmonary embolism.

Pneumonitis following radiotherapy can cause clinical symptoms in 7–8% of patients (although radiographically more frequent, ~40%). This is much more frequent following radical rather than palliative radiotherapy and presents after 2–3 months, usually with a non-productive cough, dyspnoea, and/or fever.

In certain centres, endobronchial treatment is performed for palliation of large airways obstruction by tumour, e.g. endobronchial diathermy, laser, or stenting. Complications include fever, infection, and bleeding. Stents can migrate and either block previously patent lobar bronchi or come to rest in the trachea, requiring removal.

ⓘ **Presentation with unrelated illness**

Although lung cancer survival overall is low (10–15% overall at 5 years), there are subgroups who, with appropriate treatment, can hope for a much better outlook. This must be borne in mind when making decisions about aggressive treatment (e.g. deciding on ITU admission) for other acute medical problems.

Assessment and evaluation

Important points in the history (old notes/clinic letters obviously valuable):
- Timing and nature of diagnosis.
- Known extent of disease on staging CT/PET.
- Specific anti-cancer treatments (including those planned).
- Prior local chest intervention (pleural aspiration/endobronchial intervention).
- Respiratory comorbidity.

In assessing the patient, other than the mandatory CXR, routine blood tests may provide helpful pointers as to the cause of presentation, e.g. high inflammatory markers in infection or coexisting problems such as anaemia or SIADH.

In the breathless patient with an unremarkable or unchanged CXR and little else to find, consider large airway obstruction or PE. Large airway obstruction is often missed in the patient with mild dyspnoea. Listen carefully close to the patient's mouth for stridor.

Consider pericardial effusion. Is there clinical evidence of tamponade, small QRS complexes on ECG? Has the heart enlarged on CXR?

Do not measure D-dimers; they are very non-specific and will be elevated in active cancer. If PE is suspected, request a CTPA.

An up-to-date CT scan is often needed to clarify the cause of increased or new symptoms if not readily apparent on the CXR or from routine investigations.

Management

This would be dictated by the suspected diagnosis, and would generally not be any different to the non-lung cancer patient. Early discussion with the respiratory team is important.

Specific situations
Pleural effusion
If pleural malignancy is not known, a diagnostic/therapeutic tap is best first-line management where cytological results will affect management (e.g. previously suspected limited disease and radical treatment proposed; if initial cytology negative, thoracoscopy may be needed). If presenting in a patient with more advanced disease and causing significant symptoms,

intercostal drainage with a view to pleurodesis (with talc slurry) would be reasonable first-line management.

If known malignant effusion and patient is symptomatic, current practice is for up to two attempts at intercostal drainage and talc pleurodesis before consideration of an indwelling tunnelled pleural catheter in the event of further recurrence. In good performance status patients there may be a role for first line talc pleurodesis at thoracoscopy.

Malignant large airway obstruction

Start dexamethasone (e.g. 4 mg qds/8 mg bd) and request an urgent CT scan (usually can wait until normal working hours). Refer to respiratory team for consideration of palliative radiotherapy ± endobronchial intervention.

Haemoptysis

📖 Chapter 6.

Respiratory problems in neuromuscular disease

① Introduction

A variety of neuromuscular disorders may affect the ventilatory pump at different sites (Table 37.1). Most of these disorders result in respiratory muscle weakness, which results in alveolar hypoventilation and impaired cough. Patients with known neuromuscular disease may present acutely with a presentation related to their underlying neuromuscular disease (such as infection) or occasionally in end-stage ventilatory failure.

Table 37.1 Acute and chronic neuromuscular disorders that cause ventilatory failure

Level of lesion	Acute disorders	Chronic disorders
Central nervous system	Head and spinal cord injury	Multiple sclerosis
	Stroke	Parkinson's disease
	Tetanus	Shy–Drager syndrome
Anterior horn cells	Poliomyelitis	Amyotrophic lateral sclerosis
	Rabies	Muscular atrophies
	Encephalomyelitis	Post poliomyelitis
Peripheral nerves	Guillain–Barré syndrome	Hereditary neuropathies
	Critical illness neuropathy	
	Diphtheria	
	Herpes zoster	
	Phrenic nerve injury	
	Metabolic causes	
Neuromuscular junction	Botulism	Myasthenia gravis
	Organophosphate poisoning	Lambert–Eaton syndrome
	Snake bite	
Muscles	Corticosteroid myopathy	Muscular dystrophies
	Electrolyte disorders	Myotonic dystrophy
		Acid maltase deficiency
		Mitochondrial myopathies
		Inflammatory myopathies

Assessment

Features to note from the history that suggest chronic ventilatory insufficiency

- Dyspnoea (this may be masked in patients with limb weakness).
- Early morning headaches and daytime sleepiness: due to nocturnal hypoventilation. Can develop before daytime respiratory failure.
- Orthopnoea (a feature of bilateral diaphragmatic paralysis).
- Ankle oedema due to cor pulmonale.
- Known neuromuscular diagnosis (e.g. Duchenne muscular dystrophy) or symptoms suggestive of an underlying diagnosis, such as limb weakness/swallowing difficulties.

Examination

- Chest examination may show rapid and shallow breathing with poor expansion and use of accessory muscles.
- Detailed neurological and muscular examination should be performed.
- Diaphragmatic weakness should be assessed in the supine position: results in an increase in respiratory rate; use of extrathoracic muscles and abdominal paradox may be seen.
- Look for other associated problems such as pneumonia and pleural effusion.

Acute investigations

- **CXR:** useful in looking for specific chest problems such as pneumonia or effusion. May show raised diaphragm suggesting diaphragmatic paralysis or right basal consolidation suggestive of aspiration.
- **ABGs:** the hallmarks of significant respiratory weakness are hypercapnia and hypoxaemia. Hypercapnia is a late sign and develops when respiratory muscle strength is reduced to <30% of predicted. Calculating the A–a gradient is often useful to exclude significant pulmonary disease (📖 Chapter 53).
- **PFTs:** vital capacity (VC) is reduced but not sensitive for neuromuscular disease. Serial testing of VC may be useful to assess for disease progression. Diaphragmatic weakness may be suggested by a 15% decrease in the VC on moving from upright to supine.

Specialist investigations

- **Nocturnal oximetry:** nocturnal desaturation is an early feature of ventilatory failure.
- **Respiratory muscle function:** can be assessed in a number of ways but is more specialized. Includes mouth pressures, sniff nasal inspiratory pressure, sniff transdiaphragmatic pressure, and phrenic nerve stimulation.

Treatment

Acute presentation

This depends on the underlying neurological condition and whether the patient is already in end-stage disease.

- Treat any underlying respiratory problem, most commonly bronchopneumonia.
- Oxygen therapy is vital, but keep an eye on ABGs for worsening hypercapnia and acidosis.
- Chest physiotherapy is important to clear secretions as cough reflex in these patients is often depressed.
- Avoid sedatives such as benzodiazepines and respiratory depressants such as opiates.
- Close liaison with ITU as patient may require NIV or invasive ventilation.
- Specific treatments may be helpful for some conditions such as myasthenia gravis and Guillain–Barré syndrome. Involve neurologist at early stage.
- Serial spirometry may be helpful in assessing deterioration of respiratory function.

Chronic respiratory failure and NIV

- Ventilation improves mortality and morbidity but does not alter the course of the neuromuscular disease.
- As condition progresses may need daytime support.
- Need to involve patient and relatives about choice of ventilation as neuromuscular disease will continue to progress.
- Invasive ventilation via tracheostomy may be required in some patients with bulbar muscle weakness.
- End-of-life issues and palliative care are important.

Pulmonary hypertension

⑦ Pulmonary hypertension

Pulmonary hypertension (PH) was previously classified into two categories: primary pulmonary hypertension (PPH) and secondary pulmonary hypertension, depending on the presence or absence of identifiable causes or risk factors. In 2003, PH was reclassified to categories sharing similarities in pathophysiological mechanisms, clinical presentation, and therapeutic options (WHO classification, see Table 38.1).

PH is most frequently seen as an acute admission either secondary to left heart disease or lung diseases/hypoxia; in such situations the clinical features will include those of the associated condition. PH outside these conditions is rare; this chapter will give a brief summary of clinical findings in this situation. Detailed discussion on diagnosis and management is beyond the scope of this chapter (see OHRM, Chapter 32).

Definition

Pulmonary hypertension is defined as a mean pulmonary artery pressure >25 mmHg at rest and >30 mmHg on exercise.

Presentation

- Relatively non-specific. Often a delay in diagnosis of ~3 years.
- Exertional breathlessness most common symptom.
- Angina type chest pain from right ventricular ischaemia.
- Exertional syncope.

Examination findings include:
- Low-volume pulse.
- Elevated JVP.
- Right ventricular heave.
- Loud pulmonary component of the second heart sound.
- Pansystolic murmur (tricuspid regurgitation).
- Peripheral oedema.
- Low SaO_2.

Investigations

- ABG: low $PaCO_2$ and low PaO_2.
- ECG: right ventricular hypertrophy (high specificity but low sensitivity). RBBB with anterior ST abnormalities can occur. Prominent P waves suggestive of right atrial enlargement.
- CXR: enlarged proximal pulmonary arteries, enlarged right atrium and ventricle.
- Echocardiogram: enlarged right ventricle with septal flattening. The tricuspid regurgitant jet is used to estimate pulmonary artery pressure (operator dependent).
- Right heart catheterization: confirms diagnosis. Allows the measurement of right heart pressure, cardiac output, and response to vasodilators.

Table 38.1 Classification and causes of pulmonary hypertension

1. Pulmonary arterial hypertension (PAH)

    1.1. Idiopathic (IPAH)

    1.2. Familial (FPAH)

    1.3. Associated with (APAH):

        1.3.1. Collagen vascular disease

        1.3.2. Congenital systemic-to-pulmonary shunts

        1.3.3. Portal hypertension

        1.3.4. HIV infection

        1.3.5. Drugs and toxins

        1.3.6. Other

            Thyroid disorders, glycogen storage disease, Gaucher disease, hereditary haemorrhagic telangiectasia, haemoglobinopathies, myeloproliferative disorders, splenectomy

    1.4. Associated with significant venous or capillary involvement

        1.4.1. Pulmonary veno-occlusive disease (PVOD)

        1.4.2. Pulmonary capillary haemangiomatosis (PCH)

    1.5. Persistent pulmonary hypertension of the newborn

2. Pulmonary hypertension with left heart disease

    2.1. Left-sided atrial or ventricular heart disease

    2.2. Left-sided valvular heart disease

3. Pulmonary hypertension associated with lung diseases and/or hypoxemia

    3.1. Chronic obstructive pulmonary disease

    3.2. Interstitial lung disease

    3.3. Sleep-disordered breathing

    3.4. Alveolar hypoventilation disorders

    3.5. Chronic exposure to high altitude

    3.6. Developmental abnormalities

4. Pulmonary hypertension due to chronic thrombotic and/or embolic disease

    4.1. Thromboembolic obstruction of proximal pulmonary arteries

    4.2. Thromboembolic obstruction of distal pulmonary arteries

    4.3. Non-thrombotic pulmonary embolism (tumour, parasites, foreign material)

5. Miscellaneous

    Sarcoidosis, histiocytosis X, lymphangiomatosis, compression of pulmonary vessels (adenopathy, tumour, fibrosing mediastinitis)

- Other investigations
  - Bloods including FBC, U&E, LFTs, ESR, autoimmune profile.
  - Full pulmonary function tests.
  - CTPA to look for thromboembolic disease.
  - HRCT chest to look for interstitial lung disease.

Management

Once the diagnosis is made, referral to a specialist centre is required to coordinate chronic management of this condition.

General management

- Anticoagulation: all patients with pulmonary hypertension are at risk of venous thromboembolism. Aim for INR 2–3.
- Oxygen: patient may be hypoxaemic due to combination of reduced cardiac output and ventilation/perfusion mismatch.
- Diuretics: may be useful for treatment of oedema but may reduce preload.
- Graded exercise activities: patients should be given an exercise programme.
- Vasodilator therapy: patients assessed during right heart catheterization. High-dose calcium-channel blockers such as nifedipine (80 mg/day) and diltiazem (360 mg/day) used. Less than 10% of patients benefit.
- Prostacyclins: continuous infusion of epoprostenol.
- Endothelin receptor blockers such as bosentan 125 mg bd.
- Phosphodiesterase inhibitors such as sildenafil and tadalafil.
- Digoxin may improve cardiac output.

Several surgical options can be considered, including heart lung transplant (see OHRM, Chapter 32).

End-of-life care

To improve symptoms of breathlessness, fatigue, and peripheral oedema (📖 Chapter 16).

Respiratory conditions associated with connective tissue disorders

⑦ Introduction

Pulmonary complications are common in patients with connective tissue disorders (CTDs). They can be either specific respiratory conditions related to the CTD or side effects of medication used to treat the CTD, including opportunistic infection. When a rheumatological patient presents with acute respiratory symptoms, a number of disease-specific diagnoses should be considered

① Specific respiratory conditions related to CTDs

These can predate symptoms of the CTD or develop later.

Respiratory conditions which might present acutely

Pleural effusion

- Common but often asymptomatic.
- Typically an exudate, often lymphocytic.
- Need to exclude other causes of effusion such as empyema and neoplasm (◻ Chapter 24 for approach to diagnosis and management of pleural effusion).
- If problematic may require drainage or steroids.

Acute pneumonitis

- Rare but high mortality rate.
- Presents with cough, dyspnoea, fever, and pleuritic chest pain.
- CXR shows infiltrates.
- Treatment is supportive: steroids and cytotoxics may be useful.

Organizing pneumonia

- Presents with fever, dyspnoea, and consolidation on CXR, which may be multifocal and/or flitting.
- Raised inflammatory markers.
- Mimics bacterial pneumonia but no response to antibiotics.
- Good response to steroids in >80% of cases.

Pulmonary vasculitis

- Rare in CTD; more commonly associated with pulmonary–renal syndromes (◻ Chapter 29).
- Can present with alveolar hemorrhage and haemoptysis.
- Treat with high-dose steroids and/or cytotoxics.
- Plasma exchange may be useful.

Chronic respiratory conditions

Pulmonary fibrosis

- Most common respiratory problem associated with CTD, especially rheumatoid arthritis (UIP pattern usual) and systemic sclerosis (NSIP pattern usual). For further details, see OHRM Chapter 40.
- Slowly progressive dyspnoea; bibasal fine inspiratory crackles.
- PFTs show a restrictive picture and reduced transfer factor.

Bronchiectasis

- Common; 30% of RA patients have HRCT evidence of bronchiectasis.
- More common in female seropositive patients.
- Diagnosis and management as for idiopathic bronchiectasis
  (📖 Chapter 31).

Pulmonary nodules

- Usually asymptomatic.
- May be seen as coincidental CXR finding in approximately 1% of
  patients with RA.
- Usually subpleural and can be up to several centimetres in diameter.
- Rarely cavitate; may cause haemoptysis and abscess formation.
- Cannot be differentiated from bronchial carcinoma on plain CXR
  (usually need CT thorax and biopsy).

Pulmonary hypertension

- Can develop secondary to pulmonary fibrosis.
- Systemic sclerosis can cause isolated pulmonary hypertension
  pathophysiologically similar to PPH (📖 Chapter 38).
- Presents with dyspnoea and features of right heart failure.
- Diagnosis is with echocardiography.
- Treatment is as for PPH but has better prognosis.

Obliterative bronchiolitis

- Rare complication.
- Presents with dyspnoea and hyperinflated lungs due to progressive
  irreversible airflow obstruction.
- Treat with trial of steroids but often ineffective.

① Specific respiratory conditions related to drugs used for CTDs

Methotrexate pneumonitis

- Most common life-threatening drug-induced complication seen in RA
  patients (prevalence 0.3–11%).
- Usually occurs within the first 6 months of therapy, caused by a
  hypersensitivity reaction.
- Presents acutely or subacutely with cough and dyspnoea. Fever and
  crackles in 45%.
- CXR shows bilateral, predominantly basal, interstitial infiltrates. HRCT
  thorax demonstrates ground glass change.
- Stop methotrexate and discuss case with respiratory specialist as
  differential diagnosis includes opportunistic infection and
  bronchoscopy may be required.
- High-dose corticosteroids (60 mg/day) may be beneficial.

Gold
- Can cause fever and dyspnoea with pulmonary infiltrates on CXR and CT.
- Treatment: stop the drug and start steroids. Usually reversible.

Penicillamine
Can cause obliterative bronchiolitis, hypersensitivity pneumonitis, and pulmonary–renal syndrome with alveolar haemorrhage.

① Opportunistic pulmonary infection

- Patient may be immunosuppressed by drugs or by the underlying disease.
- Often presents with non-specific symptoms of low-grade fever, cough, and dyspnoea.
- Any opportunistic organism may be involved, including TB, PCP, fungi and CMV.
- 📖 Chapter 13 for details of assessment and management.

Sickle cell disease

① Sickle cell disease

This is one of the most common inherited conditions in the world and affects predominantly people from equatorial Africa but also those of Mediterranean, Indian, and Middle-Eastern descent. It is recessively inherited and in the homozygous form (HbSS) causes a multi-organ disorder.

Pathogenesis

At times of low blood oxygenation the abnormal haemoglobin forms crystals. This changes the flexible biconcave red blood cell into rigid structures forming a sickle shape which block capillaries and cause vaso-occlusion. The vaso-occlusion occurs throughout the body and causes multi-organ damage.

Natural history

- In the UK most children are diagnosed at birth by neonatal screening.
- In countries where there is no screening, presentation is usually from 6 months and above.
- The clinical course and age of presentation is highly variable.
- The most common complications are shown in the box opposite.
- Pulmonary complications include:
  - acute chest crisis.
  - chronic sickle lung disease.
  - pulmonary hypertension.

Acute chest syndrome

- Most common cause of mortality.
- Presents with fever, chest pain, dyspnoea, and cough.
- CXR can be normal but may show infiltrates.
- Can be rapidly progressive, developing over a few hours.
- Infection is the most common precipitant, but it is also caused by hypoventilation from pain, fat embolism from bony infarction, and thrombosis.

Management

▶▶ This is a medical emergency.

- Treatment is with IV fluids, high-flow oxygen, and pain relief.
- Broad-spectrum antibiotics are often given as it is difficult to exclude infection.
- Close monitoring is required and the patient may need to be managed in an HDU or ITU setting.
- Use PaO_2 as an indicator of severity to guide management (see Table 40.1).
- Involve haematologist early as exchange transfusion may be required.
- Bronchodilators may be of benefit.
- Heparin therapy is not routinely required unless clinical suspicion of pulmonary embolism.

Box 40.1 Common complications of sickle cell disease

- Painful vaso-occlusive crisis.
- Acute chest syndrome.
- Avascular necrosis.
- Acute splenic or hepatic sequestration.
- Aplastic crisis.
- Priapism.
- Proliferative retinopathy.
- Stroke.
- Leg ulcers.
- Cholecystitis.

Table 40.1 Management of acute chest syndrome

Arterial blood gas results	Action
PaO_2 (on air) <10.5 kPa	Use 35% oxygen mask
PaO_2 (on air) <9.5 kPa	CPAP
PaO_2 (on air) <8 kPa	CPAP (discuss exchange transfusion)
PaO_2 (on air) <7.5 kPa	CPAP and exchange transfusion
If PaO_2 <7.5 kPa on oxygen	Ventilate and exchange transfusion

Chronic sickle lung disease

The incidence of chronic organ damage including chronic sickle lung disease is increasing as patients are living longer. Chronic sickle lung disease occurs secondary to an acquired vasculopathy as a result of chronic damage to the small arterioles of the lung. A history of acute chest syndrome is the most important predictor of chronic sickle lung disease but it can happen in its absence.

- Presents with progressive breathlessness.
- Can cause respiratory failure at end stage.
- CXR may be normal in the early stage but later shows features of fibrosis.
- HRCT is more sensitive and shows fibrosis.
- PFTs show features of restrictive lung disease with a decrease in lung volumes, the most sensitive early marker of chronic lung disease.
- All patients should be screened for chronic lung disease with annual PFTs.

Management

- Management is difficult and there are no randomized trials to assess the most effective treatment strategies.
- Treatment options include home oxygen, hydroxyurea, transfusion therapy, and anticoagulation.

Pulmonary hypertension

- This is common and an important cause of morbidity and mortality.
- Pathogenesis is thought to be due to haemolysis, releasing haemoglobin that acts as a nitric oxide scavenger. The deficiency in nitric oxide causes vasoconstriction and obliteration of the pulmonary vessels.
- Patients are often asymptomatic until the late stages of disease.

Management

- Patients should be referred to a tertiary pulmonary hypertension centre (📖 Chapter 38).

Sleep disordered breathing

⑦ Sleep disordered breathing

Sleep disordered breathing is a relatively new area of respiratory medicine. It encompasses two broad and sometimes overlapping groups: the first and largest is obstructive sleep apnoea (OSA), and the second is the nocturnal hypoventilatory disorders. Both require nocturnal respiratory support, usually via a nasal or face mask, although sometimes via a tracheostomy. The on-call acute physician will be consulted about patients who have sleep disordered breathing and hence should be aware of the diagnoses and the therapies.

Obstructive sleep apnoea

OSA is characterized by repeated upper airway occlusion during sleep. This is accompanied by arterial hypoxaemia and hypercapnia together with increasing respiratory effort against the occluded upper airway. The apnoea is terminated by an arousal from sleep to open the upper airway, allowing ventilation to continue. If this process is repeated many times an hour, sleep is fragmented, resulting in the characteristic symptom of OSA syndrome: excessive daytime somnolence. OSA is very effectively treated by continuous positive airway pressure (CPAP) which is delivered by a tight-fitting nasal or face mask worn during sleep. The CPAP 'splints' open the upper airway throughout the respiratory cycle, preventing the cycle of occlusion, apnoea, and arousal.

- Most patients with OSA do NOT have daytime type 2 respiratory failure and cor pulmonale. Those who do often have an overlap syndrome with another respiratory problem such as COPD.
- Patients should bring their CPAP machines into hospital to be used on the ward. Most patients can be relied upon to set them up themselves, as they do this every night at home.
- In a well person with OSA (not in ventilatory failure), CPAP is for control of daytime symptoms and can be safely omitted overnight if it is not practical to continue it.

Anaesthesia

Patients with OSA are at higher risk of anaesthetic complications. Ensure that the anaesthetist responsible for the patient is aware of the diagnosis.

- A 'difficult airway' may need a different induction technique.
- Anaesthetic, sedative, and opiate analgesic drugs cause muscle relaxation, increasing upper airway narrowing. They also blunt the respiratory drive and arousal mechanisms, worsening apnoeas.
- Extubation should be done when the patient is fully awake, preferably sitting up, with non-invasive CPAP available and appropriate staff on hand in case of a problem. Monitoring in recovery or on HDU maybe needed.

Respiratory

Presentation with cor pulmonale and ventilatory failure, i.e. 'decompensation' of OSA and overlap disorders, is discussed elsewhere (📖 Chapter 8). Therapy involves ensuring the use of CPAP or the introduction of NIV, diuretic therapy, and treating the cause of the deterioration.

Cardiovascular

CPAP is an effective therapy in acute cardiogenic pulmonary oedema in both OSA and non-OSA patients. Ensure that CPAP is continued in patients with OSA admitted with cardiogenic pulmonary oedema in addition to pharmacological therapy.

Nocturnal hypoventilation disorders

This encompasses a group of disorders in which pathology from brain-stem to respiratory muscles results in the capacity of the respiratory pump being insufficient, with resultant ventilatory failure (📖 Chapter 37, Table 37.1). They are united by worsening hypoventilation overnight, especially during REM sleep; this results in arterial hypoxaemia and hypercapnia, although without the increased respiratory effort of OSA. The arousal from these episodes results in daytime sleepiness and, as the disease progresses, chronic ventilatory failure develops.

Part of the management of these conditions is long-term NIV. Varying levels of pressure support between inspiration and expiration augment tidal volume. This improves minute ventilation, resets central hypercapnic respiratory drive, rests the respiratory muscles, and therefore lowers $PaCO_2$. The daytime symptoms are ameliorated as the arousals are prevented and the blood gases are improved even during the day when NIV is not used.

- Patients using chronic ventilatory support should be under the care of a specialist physician (usually respiratory, but in some centres the service is run by a neurologist or anaesthetist).
- Support if needed or when specific questions arise is available from the specialist unit. As well as medical input there are usually physiotherapy or nurse specialists available during the day for practical issues.

Anaesthesia

Ideally, anaesthesia should be a carefully managed elective procedure.
- As in OSA the drugs used in anaesthesia suppress ventilatory drive.
- Post-operative physiotherapy with early reintroduction of NIV is the key to avoiding respiratory complications. Elective admission to the ICU should be considered.

Respiratory

With ventilatory capacity diminished, many of these patients have limited reserve to withstand cardiorespiratory insults, such as pneumonia.
- Omission of NIV is less well tolerated than omitting CPAP in OSA and therefore, if at all possible, should not be stopped.
- Worsening respiratory failure and cor pulmonale are the usual features of decompensation.
- Treatment requires addressing the cause of deterioration and continued NIV (📖 Chapters 8 and 47).
- Ventilator settings and entrained oxygen in the acute illness may need to be changed to account for changing lung mechanics.

Intensive care

The use of home ventilatory support should not automatically preclude ICU admission. Each case should be judged on its merits with careful consideration of the underlying diagnosis, reason for deterioration, pre-morbid state, and lung function, as well as the reason for ventilation, together with patient and family wishes.

Further reading

Chapman S, Robinson G, Stradling J, West S (2005). *Oxford Handbook of Respiratory Medicine*, pp. 331–51, 597–605. Oxford University Press, Oxford.

Part 5

Practical and management issues

Airway management

Aims of airway management

- To relieve upper airway obstruction.
- To facilitate positive pressure ventilation.
- To protect respiratory tract from aspiration of gastric contents.

Upper airway obstruction is a commonly encountered emergency and is often relieved by simple basic airway manoeuvres. Although many patients will go on to require more advanced management (e.g. tracheal intubation), such procedures carry a high failure rate and should not be performed by inexperienced practitioners. However, it is still useful to have a good knowledge about advanced airway manoeuvres as it enables the non-anaesthetist to prepare some of the equipment needed and to assist during the procedure once expert help has arrived.

This chapter does not cover paediatric airway management.

☠ Upper airway obstruction

The upper airway stretches from the mouth and nose to the carina.

Level of obstruction

- Supraglottic (above vocal cords).
- Glottic (involving vocal cords).
- Infraglottic (below vocal cords).

Most sudden and acutely life threatening obstructions are supraglottic.

Causes

Functional

- Central nervous system depression (e.g. cerebrovascular accident, traumatic brain injury, metabolic, alcohol).
- Peripheral nervous and neuromuscular dysfunction (e.g. recurrent laryngeal nerve palsy, laryngospasm, Guillain–Barré syndrome).

Mechanical

- Foreign body (including vomitus).
- Oedema.
- Infection.
- Haematoma.
- Trauma.
- Burns.
- Neoplasm.
- Congenital.

Clinical signs

In a conscious patient the diagnosis is often easy. In unconscious patients a high index of suspicion, adequate exposure of the patient, and careful examination are required. A brief history from witnesses, paramedics, etc. may lead to the cause.

Complete obstruction

- Silent.
- Unable to breathe or speak despite forceful respiratory effort.
- Tracheal tug and intercostal recession.
- Hand on throat.
- Agitation and distress.
- ⚠ Emergency!
  Unless treated immediately, the patient will die within minutes.

Partial obstruction

- Noisy.
- Inspiratory stridor, gurgling, choking.
- Paradoxical chest wall movement ('see-sawing').
- Tracheal tug and intercostal recession.
- ⚠ Emergency!
  May deteriorate rapidly and progress into complete obstruction.

Airway manoeuvres

Non-invasive techniques

These are used to overcome upper airway obstruction and to maintain an open airway. They can be used in spontaneously breathing or ventilated patients.

Head tilt and chin lift

Extend the neck by placing one hand on the patient's forehead and tilting the head backwards. Use the fingers of the other hand to push the chin upwards, lifting the jaw. Do not use this technique in suspected cervical spine injury—use jaw thrust.

Jaw thrust

Place the tips of your fingers behind the angle of the jaw and pull forward. At the same time open the mouth with your thumbs.

Suction

A wide-bore sucker (e.g. Yankauer) can be used to clear the upper airway of gastric contents, blood, and saliva. It is best used in conjunction with a laryngoscope or tongue depressor to prevent pharyngeal trauma and bleeding. Conscious patients may gag and vomit.

Oropharyngeal airway (OPA)

This rigid plastic tube is easy to insert but may not be tolerated by conscious or semiconscious patients. Its length equates to the vertical distance between the angle of the jaw and the patient's incisors.

Nasopharyngeal airway (NPA)

This soft plastic tube is generally better tolerated than an oropharyngeal airway and is useful when oral access is not available (e.g. jaw clenching, trismus). Mucosal damage and bleeding are common. Its use is relatively contraindicated in base of skull fractures. Its length equates to the distance between the tip of the nose and the tragus of the ear.

Face mask

This can be used in conjunction with OPA and NPA for mouth-mask or bag–mask ventilation. Some pocket resuscitation masks have a port for the connection of oxygen. A two-handed technique is recommended for its use. The mask is held onto the face with the thumbs whilst the fingers perform a jaw thrust and pull the face into the mask.

Laryngeal mask airway (LMA)

The LMA consists of a wide bore tube and an inflatable cuff, which seals around the laryngeal inlet.

Even with little practice LMAs are relatively easy to insert and ventilation is often more efficient than through a face mask. LMAs are now widely available in hospital resuscitation kits and are being used with good results in pre-hospital care.

Problems can arise in cases of high airway resistance (e.g. severe asthma) or poor lung compliance where high inflation pressures may produce a significant leak. This may result in inadequate ventilation and gastric inflation with an increased risk of regurgitation. The LMA offers minimal protection against aspiration of gastric contents. Conscious or semiconscious patient are unlikely to tolerate this device.

Insertion

- In adults size 4 is usually used for females and size 5 for males.
- After inspecting and checking the device, lubricate the outer part of the cuff (same side as black line on tube) with water-soluble gel.
- Open the mouth and flex the neck slightly (unless suspected cervical spine injury).
- Hold the LMA like a pen and insert it into the mouth with the black line on the tube facing the patient's nose and the opening pointing towards the patient's feet.
- Guiding the mask with your index finger, push upwards and backwards to allow it to slide along the hard palate. When it reaches the posterior pharyngeal wall push slightly downwards until resistance is felt.
- Inflate the cuff with air (usually 30 ml for size 4 and 40 ml for size 5). If placed correctly the LMA should slide out by about 1–2 cm.
- Connect to a self-inflating bag and oxygen and inflate the chest. With correct placement there should be no or only minimal audible leak. Inspect and listen to the chest to confirm air entry.
- If unsuccessful or in doubt remove the LMA and oxygenate with a face mask.

Invasive techniques

Tracheal intubation

This is the 'gold standard' for securing the airway. It facilitates positive pressure ventilation, prevents air leakage even with high inflation pressures, and protects the lungs from soiling with gastric contents or other material (e.g. blood).

However, tracheal intubation, especially in an emergency situation, can be very difficult and should only be undertaken by practitioners who have been appropriately trained. In inexperienced hands the risk of unrecognized misplacement of the tube is high and can result in hypoxia and death. In conscious or semiconscious patients an emergency anaesthetic is required, which poses its own significant risks.

❶ If you are unfamiliar with tracheal intubation, call for expert help and oxygenate the patient using non-invasive techniques.

Equipment required
- Cuffed tracheal tubes: size 7.0 (internal diameter in millimetres) for females and size 8.0 for males.
- Syringe for cuff inflation.
- Laryngoscope: usually Macintosh (curved) size 3 or 4.
- Water-soluble lubricating jelly.
- Magill's forceps.
- Introducer (gum elastic bougie).
- Tape or tie to secure tube in place.
- Stethoscope.
- Suction with Yankauer attachment.
- End-tidal CO_2 detector.

Technique
- Position patient supine and flat with head in sniffing position (pillow under head and shoulders).
- Pre-oxygenate with high-flow oxygen and bag and mask.
- Standing behind the patient, hold the laryngoscope with your left hand and advance the blade along the right edge of the tongue into the pharynx. Place the tip of the blade into the vallecula between the root of the epiglottis and the base of the tongue. Now lift the laryngoscope forwards and upwards (do not tilt or touch the incisors), which pulls the epiglottis up and brings the vocal cords into view.
- Place the tube through the vocal cords and inflate the cuff.
- Confirm placement by auscultation and detection of end-tidal CO_2.

Cricoid pressure
If the patient is not adequately starved, cricoid pressure should be applied throughout the procedure until the airway is secured to prevent regurgitation of gastric contents and pulmonary aspiration. An assistant places thumb and index finger onto the cricoid cartilage and applies a pressure of 30 N (3 kg) in an anteroposterior direction.

Cannula and surgical cricothyroidotomy
These techniques should only be used in life-threatening situations in which it proves impossible to ventilate or oxygenate the patient by any of the means above. Both can have serious complications.

Cannula cricothyroidotomy

The lungs are inflated via a cannula in the cricothyroid membrane. Exhalation is passive and air has to pass through the upper airway. Allow adequate time for exhalation and abandon the procedure if the exhaled air cannot escape.

- Position the patient supine with the head slightly extended (do not overextend as this narrows the trachea).
- Identify the cricothyroid membrane between thyroid and cricoid cartilage and insert a kink-resistant cricothyroidotomy cannula through the membrane into the trachea aiming 45° caudally. Confirm correct placement by aspirating air with a 20 ml syringe attached (if not available, use a large-bore IV cannula).
- Withdraw the needle and advance the cannula.
- An assistant needs to maintain the position of the cannula to prevent kinking or displacement.
- Attach to a high-pressure ventilation system, such as a manual jet ventilation unit. Apply short bursts and observe the chest rise. Allow time for expiration.
- If this is not available, attach a high-flow oxygen supply via standard tubing and a three-way tap (all limbs open) to the cannula. Occlude the open limb with your finger for 1 second or until the chest rises adequately, then release for 3–4 seconds or until expiration complete. If no three-way tap is available, hold the oxygen tubing against the cannula for 1 second before taking it off to allow expiration.
- Abandon and convert to surgical cricothyroidotomy if ventilation fails or surgical emphysema develops.

Surgical cricothyroidotomy

Assemble a scalpel (short and round) and a small (e.g. 6 or 7 mm) cuffed tracheal or tracheostomy tube. Alternatively use a mini-tracheostomy kit.

- Identify cricothyroid membrane.
- Perform a stab incision through the skin and membrane. Enlarge incision through blunt dissection (e.g. forceps or scalpel handle).
- Use a tracheal hook for caudal traction on the cricoid cartilage.
- Insert a tracheal or tracheostomy tube and inflate cuff.
- Ventilate with a self-inflating bag.
- Confirm placement with auscultation and end-tidal CO_2 detector.
- If ventilation fails or surgical emphysema develops, abandon procedure and reassess.

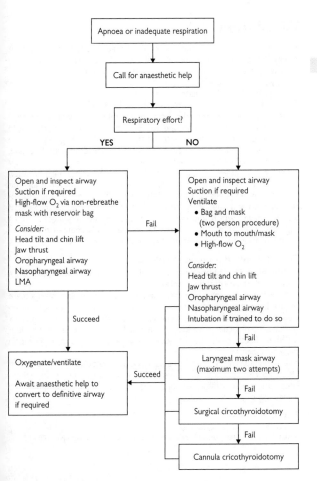

Fig. 42.1 Airway management algorithm for apnoea and inadequate respiration. NB. All airway techniques, especially tracheal intubation, LMA insertion and cricothyroidotomies, can have serious complications and should only be applied after appropriate training.

Ventilation

If a patient is apnoeic or the respiration is inadequate, despite a patent airway, artificial ventilation should be started. This can be achieved by:

- blowing into the patient's airway (mouth to mouth/nose/mask/tube).
- using a self inflatable bag.
- using a mechanical ventilator.

Whenever possible high-flow oxygen should be attached.

Ideal tidal volumes are in the region of 6–8 ml/kg body weight, which in a normal adult equates to around 400–600 ml. This is often not possible to measure and as a guide each inflation should be large enough to produce visible chest movement and should be delivered over 1 second. The rate should be 12–16 inflations/minute.

Ensure the airway is patent at all times and avoid high inflation pressures as well as excessive tidal volumes, as they will force air into the oesophagus, causing gastric distension. This increases the risk of regurgitation and pulmonary aspiration and may also lead to splinting of the diaphragm, which impedes lung compliance and ventilation. During bag–mask ventilation a two-person technique greatly reduces the risk of gastric inflation and improves the effectiveness of ventilation.

Effects of ventilation on circulation

Positive-pressure ventilation has many effects on cardiovascular physiology, a few of which are described below.

As intrathoracic pressure increases, venous return and preload are reduced, leading to a fall in cardiac output. This response may be exaggerated in hypovolaemic patients. However, in patients with cardiac pulmonary oedema, the reduction in preload and afterload may improve cardiac function.

Other effects are due to changes in partial pressure of CO_2. Hypocapnia causes an increase in systemic vascular resistance, afterload, and myocardial workload. This may lead to a fall in cardiac output and a reduction in blood flow to vital organs. Hypercapnia causes vasodilatation and stimulates sympathetic activity, resulting in an increase in cardiac output and a higher risk of arrhythmias.

Further information

Difficult Airway Society: www.das.uk.com
Allman K, Wilson I (2006). *Oxford Handbook of Anaesthesia*. Oxford University Press, Oxford.

Tracheostomy

Indications

- Upper airway obstruction.
- Prolonged ventilation.
- Protection against pulmonary aspiration.
- Tracheobronchial toilet.
- Major head & neck surgery.
- Aids earlier weaning from a ventilator.

Tracheostomies are commonly used in ICUs if prolonged ventilation is anticipated. However, there is no consensus on when they should be performed. The timing ranges from early (4–7 days) to late (10–21 days). Tracheostomy tubes are more comfortable and better tolerated than translaryngeal tubes, reducing sedation requirements. Furthermore, they facilitate tracheal suctioning, minimize dead space, and decrease the resistance to breathing.

Management of long-term indwelling tracheostomies is beyond the scope of this book.

Priority

Elective

The majority of tracheostomies are performed as elective procedures in the operating theatre or ICU.

Urgent

Occasionally tracheostomies are performed under local anaesthesia or careful sedation in patients with upper airway obstruction, in whom conventional intubation is thought to be very difficult or impossible.

Emergency

Performing a formal tracheostomy takes some time and therefore is unsuitable in a true airway emergency with worsening hypoxaemia. In such a scenario cannula or surgical cricothyroidotomy should be employed instead.

Procedure

The tracheostomy is usually sited below the first tracheal ring. This can be done as a surgical procedure ('open' or 'conventional') or as a percutaneous dilatation technique.

Percutaneous tracheostomies can be performed at the bedside on ICU. A cannula is inserted into the trachea percutaneously. A guidewire is then passed through the cannula and the latter is removed. An introducer and dilator are then fed over the guidewire into the trachea to form an opening large enough to admit a tracheostomy tube.

Anatomy

- The larynx consists of three large unpaired cartilages (epiglottis, thyroid, and cricoid) and six smaller paired cartilages (arytenoids, cuneiforms and corniculates).

- The cricothyroid membrane covers the gap between the thyroid and cricoid cartilage.
- The trachea extends from the lower border of the cricoid cartilage to the carina (15 cm in an adult). It has approximately 20 C-shaped cartilaginous rings, which are deficient posteriorly. The trachealis muscle forms the posterior border of the trachea.
- Motor, sensory, and autonomic innervation of the larynx and trachea come from branches of the vagus nerve (superior and recurrent laryngeal nerves) and from branches of the middle cervical ganglion.
- Large vessels (including the aortic arch) and nerves, as well as the vascular thyroid gland, lie in close proximity to the trachea.

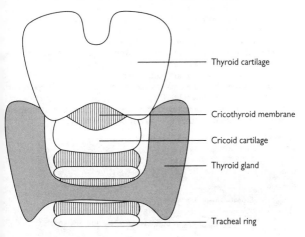

Thyroid cartilage

Cricothyroid membrane

Cricoid cartilage

Thyroid gland

Tracheal ring

Fig. 43.1 Anatomy.

Changes in physiology

- The airway resistance decreases as the upper airway is bypassed.
- Inspired air is not warmed and humidified, as it does not pass through the nose and mouth. This results in increased mucus production and altered colonization of the upper airways.
- Cough is severely impaired or impossible, as the patient is unable to produce the high intrathoracic pressures required for coughing, which are usually achieved by straining against a closed glottis.
- The normal swallowing mechanism is impaired because of splinting of the larynx.
- Patients are unable to speak unless the cuff is deflated or special attachments (e.g. speaking valve, fenestrated tube) are used.
- The sense of smell is potentially impaired because of reduced airflow through the nasal passages.

Tracheostomy tubes and attachments

A variety of tube shapes, lengths, and diameters and tube attachments are available.

- *Fixed or variable length*: variable (adjustable flange) tubes are used if there is a concern that the tube may not reach the trachea. This can be the case in patients with increased pre-tracheal space (e.g. obesity, goitre) or other deformities.
- *Cuffed or uncuffed*: uncuffed tubes are used to overcome upper airway obstruction or to facilitate tracheal suctioning of secretions in patients who do not need ventilation and are not at risk of aspiration. Tubes used for ventilation are usually cuffed.
- *Single or double (with or without an inner tube)*: the inner tube can be removed for cleaning, whilst the outer tube remains *in situ*.
- *Fenestrated or non-fenestrated*: fenestrated tubes have a series of holes in their outer curvature, through which expiratory airflow is directed to pass through the vocal cords to aid phonation. The holes can be blocked off with a non-fenestrated inner tube.
- *Speaking valves*: these are one-way valves which are placed on the outer end of the tracheostomy tube. They allow air to be inhaled but close on exhalation, directing the airflow through the vocal cords. Cuffed tubes have to be deflated and the upper airway needs to be patent.

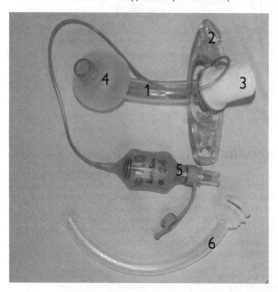

Fig. 43.2 Tracheostomy tubes and attachments: (1) outer cannula; (2) flange/neck plate; (3) 15 mm adaptor; (4) cuff; (5) pilot balloon; (6) inner cannula.

Complications

Immediate (<24 hours)
- Haemorrhage.
- Injury to trachea, larynx, and neighbouring structures.
- Air embolism.
- Displacement of tube and loss of airway.

Early (1–14 days)
- Subcutaneous emphysema, pneumothorax, and pneumomediastinum.
- Tube displacement and blockage.
- Wound infection.
- Tracheal necrosis and tracheomalacia.
- Secondary haemorrhage.

Late (>2 weeks)
- Haemorrhage due to erosion into large vessels.
- Tracheo-oesophageal fistula.
- Laryngeal or tracheal stenosis.

General considerations

- ⚠ Call for anaesthetic and ENT help early.
- ⚠ Changing of tracheostomy tubes is associated with considerable risks, particularly in an emergency situation. It should only be performed by appropriately trained and experienced practitioners, who have the knowledge and skills required to manage the airway if the tube exchange fails.
- ⚠ In a recently fashioned tracheostomy (<7 days) a tract has not yet formed and the stoma may close quickly after the tube has been removed. Percutaneous dilatational stomas may be more prone to collapse than surgical stomas. Early replacement of a tracheostomy tube can be very difficult and carries a high risk of creating a false passage. Positive-pressure ventilation into a false passage can result in rapid development of pneumothorax, pneumomediastinum, and subcutaneous emphysema of neck, larynx, and pharynx. This can render further airway management and ventilation impossible.
- ▶ Equipment for an emergency tube change should be readily available for each patient with a tracheostomy. This should include:
  - tracheostomy tubes (same size and one size smaller).
  - tracheal dilator.
  - bougie.
  - stitch cutters.
  - self-inflatable bag and mask.
  - oxygen source and tubing.
  - syringe.
  - stethoscope.
  - suction.

☠ **Specific problems and emergencies**

⚠ Call for anaesthetic and ENT help early.

Poor cuff seal

This may be due to a lack of air in the cuff, a cuff leak, or poor tube alignment.

- Check the alignment of head and neck and bring them into midline.
- Check the position of the tube; it may be too short and it may need changing.
- Inflate the cuff, taking care not to over-inflate it; check the cuff pressure.

Subcutaneous emphysema

This can be caused by a poor cuff seal, tube misalignment, or partial tube displacement.

⚠ It may compromise the airway rapidly.

Tube displacement

This is a medical emergency.

⚠ *Partial displacement*

If the chest is expanding well and there is good air entry on auscultation, the tube is probably still in the trachea.

- Deflate the cuff and carefully reposition the tube before re-inflating.

⚠ *Complete displacement*

If chest expansion and breath sounds are absent, the tube is not in the trachea and may be compressing it.

- Deflate the cuff and remove the tube immediately.
- If the patient is breathing spontaneously and there is now good air entry and sufficient airflow across the stoma, administer oxygen via the stoma (not via the face). If this is not possible, cover the stoma with an occlusive dressing and deliver oxygen via a face mask.
- If ventilation is required, cover the stoma and ventilate via the upper airway as in a non-tracheostomy patient (📖 Chapter 42).
- Prepare for conventional translaryngeal intubation.

Obstructed tracheostomy tube

This presents with stridor and difficulty breathing. Common causes are as follows.

- *Sputum or blood*: remove and clean the inner tube; suction through the tube with a sterile suction catheter. The tube may need changing.
- *Poor alignment within trachea*: Check the head and neck alignment and carefully reposition tube.
- *Herniated cuff*: Often helped by carefully deflating the cuff. The tube will need changing.

Oxygen therapy

⚙ Oxygen therapy

Prompt and correct use of oxygen therapy underpins the management of nearly all respiratory emergencies. Time spent familiarizing yourself with local policy and equipment can prove invaluable in the emergency situation.

Principles

The underlying goal of oxygen therapy is to deliver the tissues with an adequate supply to fulfil their metabolic requirement. Key to this process is the delivery of oxygen (DO_2) equation:

$$DO_2 = \text{cardiac output} \times \text{oxygen content}$$

$$\text{oxygen content} = Hb \times SaO_2 \times 1.36 +$$

$$(PaO_2 \text{ dissolved in plasma} \times 0.023)$$

Oxygen is carried almost entirely by haemoglobin. The amount of oxygen dissolved in plasma contributes <2% which explains why haemoglobin saturation, haemoglobin concentration, and the cardiac output are all important to target in the management of the critically ill patient rather than simply aiming for a PaO_2.

- In the emergency setting oxygen therapy should always be considered in the context of the DO_2 and hence as part of a cardiorespiratory resuscitation plan.

Worked example

Critically ill patient with Hb 10 g/dL, PaO_2 8.0 kPa, and SpO_2 92%.
One litre of blood contains

$$10 \times 0.92 \times 1.36 \times 1\ 0\ \text{(convert litres)} = 125\ ml\ O_2/L.$$

If the cardiac output is 4 L/min,

$$DO_2 = 4 \times 125 = 500\ ml\ O_2/min.$$

↑ FiO_2 to increase SpO_2 to 97%:

$$DO_2 = 10 \times 0.97 \times 1.36 \times 10 = 131.9 \times 4 = 527\ ml\ O_2/min.$$

However, if the cardiac output is increased to 5,

$$DO_2 = 125 \times 5 = 625\ ml\ O_2/min.$$

In this example, increasing the cardiac output has increased oxygen delivery by 25%, whereas just increasing SaO_2 led to a 5% increase.

Combining increases in FiO_2 with adequate resuscitation should enable optimal tissue oxygen delivery.

Table 44.1 Oxygen delivery systems

Delivery system	Details	FiO$_2$	Comments
Reservoir bag	Mask with bag below	10–15 L provides ~0.8	First line for resuscitation. Start by inflating bag by pressing on valve. Must be fully inflated.
Hudson mask	Simple mask	5–8 L gives 0.5–0.6	Often used as 'default mask' but neither high flow nor controlled.
Venturi mask	Coloured valve system	Flow as advised on valve. FiO$_2$ is written on valve	System of choice for the hypoxic patient requiring controlled therapy. If remains hypoxic FiO$_2$ is not increased by increasing flow rate. The valve needs to be changed.
Nasal cannulae	Prong delivered	Not known	Ensure fitted correctly. FiO$_2$ dependent on flow rate and breathing pattern including respiratory rate and degree of mouth breathing. Not for sole use in emergency. Can be used in combination with other delivery systems.
CPAP	Tight-fitting face mask with special delivery system	>0.8 with PEEP	📖 Chapter 47. Useful in selected patients with significant hypoxia, e.g. LVF, pneumonia.

What is 'controlled' oxygen therapy?

A controlled system is one that permits the best degree of control over FiO$_2$. No system is perfect but, for example, a Venturi valve mask allows delivery of a prescribed FiO$_2$. In contrast, the amount of oxygen delivered by nasal cannulae varies depending upon the respiratory rate and degree of mouth breathing.

Practice: using oxygen in respiratory emergencies

Not all respiratory emergencies require acute oxygen therapy. However, if significant hypoxia is apparent or suspected proceed as below.

- The first priority in an emergency should be to **check that the airway and breathing** is adequate to 'deliver' oxygen (i.e. ABC).
- Next, commence high-flow oxygen therapy. Use a reservoir bag initially; this provides the maximal FiO_2 at high inspiratory rates; which often exceed the 15 L provided by hospital wall oxygen outlet. Ensure that the reservoir bag is inflated.
- If the patient is known to be oxygen sensitive then deliver oxygen by a controlled system and aim for a saturation that is estimated to be 'normal for the patient' (see box below).

- In the emergency setting it is often unclear if a patient is 'sensitive' to oxygen (e.g. COPD in A & E)
- If chronic lung disease is suspected, aim for an oxygen saturation between 85% and 90%
- Therapy adjustments can be made when further clinical information and ABG results are available.

- Be very careful reducing oxygen in the narcosed hypercarbic patient, e.g. a COPD patient who has been given uncontrolled excess oxygen in ambulance transit and arrives unconscious. Reducing FiO_2 quickly may precipitate cardiac arrest because of the combination of reduced FiO_2 and poor ventilation. Consider short course NIV or, if not available, try respiratory support with Ambubag after discussion with the intensive care team.
- Clearly communicate rationale for choice of oxygen delivery system and flow rate to clinical team.
- Document ongoing management strategy in notes and prescribe oxygen on the drug chart. In emergency situations, because oxygen requirements fluctuate it is probably more effective to spend time discussing plan with team and reviewing the patient regularly.

If the patient is oxygen sensitive consider recording this in the hypersensitivity section of the drug chart.

How much oxygen should be given?

- The aim is to provide an adequate supply for tissue oxygenation.
- Patients with chronic respiratory disorders have often 'adapted' to lower baseline saturations. This may be with or without chronic hypercapnia. Look for clues to help decide if this could be the case:
  - History: the underlying diagnosis and severity (FEV_1), use of home oxygen (has a doctor told them to use it for >15 hours/day? Usually LTOT patients have been assessed and should have a PaO_2 <7.3 kPa when stable). Previous use of NIV/ventilation.
  - Examination: respiratory rate may be useful, e.g. if they feel well and RR normal with SaO_2 86%.
  - Investigation: perhaps most helpful. Search old notes for previous SaO_2/ABG, especially on discharge or in clinic. Is there evidence of polycythaemia?
  - Look at the base excess and bicarbonate: if elevated, suggests compensation for chronic hypercapnia.
- If it seems likely that the patient is chronically hypoxic secondary to chronic lung disease, then target oxygen saturations to 85–90% and document in notes and on oxygen prescription chart (if used). Use clinical response and other markers of tissue oxygenation (e.g. lactate) to ensure adequate therapy.

Oxygen in emergencies: errors to look out for!

- Check tubing from bag/mask is attached to oxygen outlet (not uncommon to find it attached to air outlet in the haste of the moment).
- Acutely hypoxic patient: oxygen flow rate turned up high on venturi mask (valve means effective FiO_2 no greater) or nasal cannulae (not effective).
- 'Non-rebreathe' mask: ensure reservoir bag inflated at onset. Press on valve above bag (the bag provides a sump of oxygen for the high inspiratory flow rate generated).

Further reading

Oxford Handbook of Respiratory Medicine.
Leach RM, Treacher DF (2002) Basic concepts of oxygen delivery. *Thorax* **57**, 170–7.

Heliox

Heliox

Introduction

Helium–oxygen (heliox) mixtures were first described in the 1930s for the management of respiratory emergencies. In the last 20 years heliox has gained more widespread use. It has a role in the temporary management of upper airway obstruction and there is renewed interest in its use in acute asthma and COPD in both spontaneously breathing and mechanically ventilated patients.

Basics

Helium is a colourless, tasteless, insoluble, and non-toxic gas. It does not react with body tissues. Its benefits in acute respiratory care derive from its low density and viscosity compared with oxygen and nitrogen.

- Lower viscosity improves air flow in laminar flow situations:
  - flow α 1/viscosity
- Lower density improves air when turbulent flow occurs:
  - flow^2 α 1/density
- Lower density lowers the Reynold's number making laminar air flow more likely in a given situation.

This means that air flow will be increased in a tube even if the driving pressure remains the same, or that the same flow rate can be achieved with a lower driving pressure, i.e. a lower work of breathing. In a situation when airway resistance has increased, e.g. acute bronchospasm, these improvements are highly desirable.

The lower density also accounts for the improved flow for less respiratory effort through an orifice. Upper airway narrowing is the clinical scenario in which heliox is best known (pp. 259).

Heliox is usually a 70:30 mixture of helium and oxygen. It is thought that the improved flow dynamics require an FiHe of at least 0.6.

Upper airway obstruction

- The most common indication for heliox; most A&Es have it available in their resuscitation areas.
- It is an aid to management of upper airway obstruction alongside definitive care. It may obviate the need for intubation or allow it to happen in a more controlled setting.

COPD

The physical properties of helium could make it an attractive therapeutic manoeuvre for patients not responding to initial aggressive therapy. However, this is not clear cut. Some argue that COPD is a small airways disease where airflow is laminar, and heliox is less effective as its effects are predominantly density related.

A Cochrane review of heliox in COPD found that insufficient evidence exists to recommend it at present. NIV should remain the preferred option if medical therapy is not adequate. If heliox is available, and NIV is either not tolerated or is unavailable, then it could be used if endotracheal intubation is not suitable.

Asthma

There is no evidence supporting the use of heliox in asthma. Indeed, there are concerns that its use could be deleterious. The ability to deliver enough oxygen is the main concern, plus the possibility that it may delay endotracheal intubation.

Summary

- Heliox improves flows in laminar and turbulent flow situations and reduces the work of breathing whilst the patient is breathing the mixture, but its effects do not last long once it is removed.
- It has a clear role in temporary management of upper airway obstruction.
- It has theoretical benefits in both asthma and COPD. However, this is not proven and it should not be used in standard practice in preference to more longstanding therapies.

Further reading

Colebourn C, Barber V, Young JD (2007). Use of helium–oxygen mixture in adults presenting with acute exacerbations of asthma and COPD: a systematic review. *Anaesthesia* **62**, 34–42.

Rodrigo G, Pollack C, Rodrigo C, Rowe B, Walters EH (2003). Heliox for treatments of exacerbations of COPD. *Cochrane Database Systematic Review*.

Nebulizers

Nebulizers

Nebulizers allow the administration of drugs by generating suspensions of particles. They have assumed a central role in the management of patients with acute airways obstruction. However, it should be remembered that most nebulized medication never actually reaches the lung.

Principles and application

- Nebulizer therapy is not an efficient method of administering therapy. Particles are usually either too large or too small to reach the target area (in the acute setting it is estimated that active drug delivery can be as low as 10–20%). Recent evidence suggests inhalers ± spacing devices are equally, if not more, effective even in the emergency setting.
- In hospital, nebulizers are usually driven by gas or oxygen from the wall outlet supply. In nearly all circumstances use oxygen. To optimize drug delivery it is important that the supply is run at a flow rate of 6 L/minute. If the patient is hypoxic at this flow rate, use nasal cannulae with oxygen simultaneously.
- There is often concern regarding the use of oxygen to drive nebulizers in patients with COPD. It is unlikely that the patient will deteriorate during the course of a supervised nebulized treatment. However, if there is concern and the patient is hypoxic, then use oxygen via nasal cannulae and air to drive the nebulizer (at 6 L/minute).
- Consider changing to inhalers as soon as possible in the hospital admission. Evidence supports the efficacy of inhalers in the acute setting and early prescription allows more time to educate and check inhaler technique.
- Nebulizers for outpatient use should only be prescribed by those with specialist knowledge. The BTS issue clear guidelines (see link below).

For in-depth background regarding the science and appropriate use of nebulizer therapy – see guideline at: http://www.brit-thoracic.org.uk/

Nebulized therapies

The majority of these therapies are novel and/or specialized. It is always advisable to check local protocol before considering novel therapies.

- **Antibiotics** This route of administration has been successfully used in patients with bronchiectasis and cystic fibrosis. e.g. colistin sulphate (Colomycin®), tobramycin and gentamicin. Some antibiotics can precipitate acute bronchospasm.
- **Saline** Saline nebules are thought to free secretions and improve mucus clearance. There is limited evidence of efficacy. One study found a beneficial role as an adjunct to physiotherapy, and another found mild improvements in dyspnoea ratings but no improvement in lung function (in COPD). Nebulized 7% saline has recently been shown to have beneficial effects on lung function in cystic fibrosis.
- **DNAse** This therapy is widely used as part of the long-term management of cystic fibrosis patients. There are also reports of successful use in life-threatening asthma refractory to conventional treatment.
- **Acetylcysteine** This if often used to reduce sputum viscosity and ease secretion clearance. There are mixed reports of efficacy and it should be remembered that its molecular structure is affected by high levels of inspired oxygen.
- **Magnesium** A recent trial demonstrated the efficacy of 2.5 ml of isotonic magnesium as an adjuvant to salbutamol in the treatment of acute severe asthma. Adverse effects have been reported when magnesium is inadequately diluted. Further evidence is awaited.

Non-invasive ventilation

☼ Non-invasive ventilation

Non-invasive ventilation (NIV) refers to the delivery of ventilatory support via the upper airway using a face or nasal mask. In this chapter NIV refers to non-invasive positive pressure ventilation; negative pressure ventilation (e.g. external cuirass) is not used in the acute setting and will not be discussed. Ventilators can be either pressure or volume controlled, but bi-level pressure support ventilators are by far the most commonly used.

Continuous positive airway pressure (CPAP) is not generally considered to be ventilatory support but is indicated in the acute management of specific clinical scenarios to improve oxygenation.

Bi-level positive airway pressure (BiPAP)

Mechanism of action

The aim of NIV is to decrease the work of breathing, improving alveolar ventilation whilst resting the respiratory muscles. The inspiratory pressure delivered provides increased ventilation to help eliminate carbon dioxide, whilst the expiratory pressure provides improved alveolar ventilation (by preventing the pressure-related collapse of small airways) and recruits under-ventilated lung so improving oxygenation.

Indications

- Patients with an acute exacerbation of COPD in whom a respiratory acidosis (pH <7.35) persists despite maximal medical treatment on controlled oxygen therapy.
- Acute on chronic hypercapnic ventilatory failure due to chest wall deformity or neuromuscular disease.
- Decompensated obstructive sleep apnoea, particularly if acidotic.

NIV is used in a variety of other settings on the ICU (e.g. acute respiratory distress syndrome, acute pneumonia with hypoxaemia) where tracheal intubation can occur if NIV fails. NIV should not be used for these conditions outside the ICU (unless it has been agreed the patient is not appropriate for ICU transfer).

NIV should not be used in acute asthma.

Absolute contraindications

- Facial trauma or burns.
- Vomiting.
- Fixed upper airway obstruction.
- Undrained pneumothorax.

A chest drain should be inserted to treat pneumothorax prior to starting NIV.

Relative contraindications

In some patients NIV is used as the ceiling of treatment, in which case it may be started despite the presence of one or more of the following.

- Consolidation on CXR.
- Haemodynamic instability.
- Confusion or agitation.
- Excessive secretions.
- Severe hypoxaemia or acidosis.
- Inability to protect airway.

Factors predicting success

These include younger age, lower APACHE scores, and less severe blood gas parameters. Those who are able to cooperate and coordinate better with the machine also have better outcomes.

Setting up NIV

Patients should be on maximal medical therapy and controlled oxygen and fit the criteria as outlined above.

Prior to starting NIV, the management plan in the event of treatment failure should be discussed and documented in the notes: either to proceed to intubation and ventilation, or as a ceiling of treatment and for medical management.

- Explain to the patient the use of the machine and the mask.
- Select a mask that will fit the patient.
- Set up the ventilator: usual starting pressures are IPAP 10 and EPAP 4, with a back-up breath rate of 10–15.
- Ensure that a bacterial filter is included in circuit.
- Commence NIV holding the mask in place for the first few minutes to allow the patient to become used to it.
- Secure the mask with head straps.
- Monitor pulse oximetry.
- Entrain oxygen if required—the closer to the mask the better. Aim for oxygen saturations of 85–90%.
- Monitor respiratory rate, blood pressure, and heart rate.
- Repeat ABGs in 1 hour.

Monitoring

- Conscious level.
- Patient comfort.
- Chest wall motion.
- Accessory muscle use.
- Coordination of respiration with the ventilator.
- Respiratory rate.
- Heart rate.
- Oxygen saturation.
- Repeat ABGs at 1 hour; repeat at 4 hours if not improving.

Treatment failure

This can occur because of a failure of the gases to improve, an inability for the patient to tolerate NIV, a deterioration in the patient's general condition, or a development of new symptoms.

- Ensure optimal medical treatment of COPD.
- Confirm that all prescribed treatment is being administered (there should be a break in NIV to deliver nebulizers if they cannot be given simultaneously).
- Consider chest physiotherapy to alleviate sputum retention.
- Check that ventilator and circuit are set up correctly.
- Exclude any complications such as pneumothorax or aspiration, or complication of associated comorbidity.
- If $PaCO_2$ remains elevated, consider the following.
  - Too much oxygen.
  - Excessive leakage from mask: check mask fit or change type of mask.
  - Exclude rebreathing: check expiratory valve is patent or increase EPAP.
  - Ensure patient is synchronizing with the ventilator and ventilation is adequate: adjust rate and/or I:E ratio. Increase IPAP if ventilation inadequate.

If the above are not an issue or corrected and $PaCO_2$ remains high, consider increasing IPAP.

If PaO_2 remains low, consider increasing oxygen or increasing EPAP.

Other uses of BiPAP

Cystic fibrosis/bronchiectasis

NIV is often used successfully for acute exacerbations associated with acidosis and hypercapnia, particularly in end-stage disease where this may be the ceiling of treatment. Its use is sometimes limited by excessive secretions.

Weaning in ICU

NIV has been used successfully to wean in the ICU setting, with some studies showing reduced intubation time, reduced ICU stay, and reduced incidence of ventilator-associated pneumonia.

Cardiogenic pulmonary oedema

NIV has not been shown to be superior to CPAP.

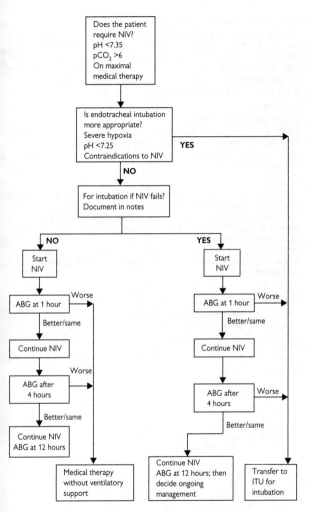

Fig. 47.1 Algorithm for setting up NIV.

Continuous positive airway pressure (CPAP)

CPAP is used in those with acute respiratory failure (type 1 respiratory failure) to correct hypoxaemia. It improves oxygenation by increasing mean airway pressure, thus increasing ventilation to collapsed areas of lung, recruiting under-ventilated areas of lung, and thereby correcting ventilation–perfusion mismatch and shunting. It also reduces inspiratory work, decreasing the work of breathing.

Uses of CPAP

Cardiogenic pulmonary oedema

CPAP has been shown to be an effective treatment in pulmonary oedema for patients who remain hypoxic despite maximal medical therapy. A number of randomized controlled studies showed a reduction in intubation rates and a reduced mortality.

Pneumonia

CPAP has been used in the treatment of severe community-acquired pneumonia as well as in the treatment of pneumocystis pneumonia in the immunocompromised, where patients remain hypoxic despite maximal medical therapy. CPAP improves oxygenation, reduces respiratory rate, and reduces dyspnoea.

Ideally, CPAP should be used in an HDU/ICU setting for these patients where intubation would be required in the event of treatment failure with CPAP.

Obstructive sleep apnoea

The most common use for CPAP is in the long-term management of obstructive sleep apnoea, where it acts as an upper airway 'splint' to eliminate apnoeic episodes.

Further reading

BTS guidelines on NIV and acute respiratory failure. Available online at: www.brit-thoracic.org.uk

Intensive care referral

:*: Intensive care medicine

Intensive care medicine is the branch of medicine that deals with acute organ failure requiring invasive supportive therapies. It involves patient care in many settings, and the more general term 'critical care' is often preferred. Very often several organs are failing at the same time. Drugs and mechanical support are now available for multiple organ systems, the oldest of which is mechanical ventilation for respiratory failure.

The two main respiratory reasons for ICU admission are hypoxaemic and/or hypercapnia respiratory failure which have failed to respond to ward care. It is not possible to be prescriptive about whom to admit to the ICU and when to admit them. However, certain principles apply and, if followed, will make for fruitful discussion with intensive care doctors and effective patient care.

Involve ICU early

Many patients admitted to ICU, or suffering a cardiac arrest in hospital, show physiological signs of deterioration for hours and days prior to this event. Early warning scoring systems have been developed and validated to help identify the potential problem patient. Most ICUs now run some form of outreach service to help advise and support the ward staff caring for such patients. It should enable the intensive care team to monitor patients and then transfer to the ICU if and when needed, hopefully maximizing the use of a scarce resource.

Ensure early resuscitation and maximum therapy

The early resuscitation of the unwell patient offers the potential to make a difference to outcome. This approach is best known through 'early goal-directed therapy'. The Surviving Sepsis Campaign is an attempt to improve the early care of patients with sepsis. Before speaking to the ICU, ensure that all possible care has been initiated on the ward or in the ED.

Realize what ICU can offer

Remember that intensive care medicine offers organ support and high levels of nursing care whilst the patient either recovers by themselves (e.g. after surgery) or responds to therapy (e.g. antibiotics for pneumonia). If neither of these options is likely, intensive care may merely prolong death.

ICU interventions have risks attached to them and deleterious consequences. Indeed, much of the benefit of NIV in COPD is in avoiding endotracheal intubation with its subsequent risks of ventilator-associated pneumonia.

Consider comorbidities

The best that any patient can hope for is to return to their premorbid level of function. Patients with multiple comorbidites, pre-existing organ dysfunction, and poor functional status are likely to have a poor outcome to their ICU stay.

COPD

COPD patients requiring NIV should have a clear plan regarding ceiling of therapy (📖 Chapter 47). There is often a nihilistic approach to invasive ventilation for COPD, although published data from the Intensive Care National Audit and Research Centre (ICNARC) suggest that patients with single organ failure, good functional status, lack of other organ dysfunction (including poor nutritional status), and a reversible disease process have a survival to discharge of 70%. This is comparable with many conditions for which the admission to ICU is not debated. Age and FEV_1 should not be used in isolation when assessing suitability. Functional status, BMI, oxygen requirements when stable, comorbidities, and previous admissions to the ICU should also be considered.

Convalescence

A medical patient admitted to the ICU is likely to have a prolonged hospital admission, including tracheostomy to facilitate weaning from ventilatory support. Following discharge from the ICU they often need high levels of ongoing care and will require convalescence and rehabilitation. Return to premorbid function may not occur, and even in those in whom it does, it can take many months and even years.

Discussion with patient and relatives

Given all of the above, admission to the ICU is often the only option for patients. If time allows, discussion of the risks and benefits should be undertaken with the patient and their family. For many people the reality of ICU is not something they would wish, and the use of palliative care techniques may be the best option. These discussions may be outside the experience or competency of the ward doctor. If needed, the ICU team should be involved to discuss these issues with the family even if ICU care is not a realistic option.

Mechanical ventilation

This refers to ventilation via an endotracheal tube or tracheostomy to enable the delivery of high inspired fractions of oxygen, effective PEEP, and control of tidal volume and respiratory rate to improve the clearance of CO_2.

- *Pressure controlled ventilation*: tidal volume is determined by preset pressures and respiratory system compliance.
- *Volume controlled ventilation*: a preset tidal volume is delivered and the airway pressures are then a consequence of the respiratory mechanics.

The use of lung protective ventilation with low tidal volumes, limiting plateau pressures, and consequent permissive hypercapnia has been shown to reduce ventilator-induced lung injury and improve survival in ARDS.

Most patients on ICU have some form of 'partial' ventilatory support; they are sedated but not paralysed and do some or most of the work of breathing themselves. They trigger the ventilator themselves at a time determined by their own respiratory drive and then receive a level of pressure support to help produce an effective tidal volume and overcome the work of breathing of the airway. This helps to reduce muscle wasting and aids with the weaning process.

Further reading

McQuillan P et al. (1998). Confidential inquiry into quality of care before admission to intensive care. *BMJ* **316**, 1854–8.

Rivers E et al. (2001). Early goal directed therapy in the treatment of severe sepsis and septic shock. *N Engl J Med* **345**, 1368–77.

Wildman M et al. (2005). Case mix and outcomes for admissions to UK adult, general critical care units with COPD: a secondary analysis of the ICNARC case mix programme database. *Crit Care*, **9**, S38–48.

Herridge M et al. (2003). One year outcome in survivors of ARDS. *N Engl J Med* **348**, 683–93.

The ARDS Network (2000). Ventilation with lower tidal volumes as compared with traditional tidal volumes for acute lung injury and the adult respiratory distress syndrome. *N Engl J Med* **342**, 1301–8.

Pre-operative assessment

⑦ Pre-operative assessment

A thorough pre-operative assessment includes taking a history, performing a physical examination, studying clinic letters and previous anaesthetic charts, and collating investigation results. The information gathered enables the physician to quantify peri-operative risks (e.g. respiratory, cardiac, etc) and allows optimization of the patient's treatment and planning of management options. Risks can then be discussed with the patient for best possible informed consent.

This chapter outlines the basics of pre-operative assessment for patients with respiratory disease but does not claim to be complete. For detailed information a formal textbook should be consulted.

Peri-operative respiratory function

Several factors play a role in the development of respiratory complications peri-operatively.

Patient factors
- Pre-existing respiratory disease.
- Other significant comorbidities, especially cardiovascular disease.
- Smoking.
- Obesity.
- Age.

Surgical factors
- Upper abdominal and thoracic surgery (reluctance to cough → development of atelectasis and sputum retention).
- Prolonged surgery.

Anaesthetic factors
General anaesthesia leads to several changes in respiratory physiology.
- Relaxation of muscles → atelectasis in dependent areas.
- ↓ FRC → prone to hypoxaemia.
- ↑ Closing volume encroaching on FRC → prone to hypoxaemia.
- ↓ Response to hypoxaemia, hypercarbia and acidosis.
These changes can last from a few hours to several days postoperatively.

History

Ascertain and document information about the following facts:
- History of dyspnoea.
- Ability to lie flat and exercise tolerance.
- Cough, sputum, recent infection.
- Cigarette consumption.
- Previous hospital admissions, operations, ICU admissions.
- Type of treatment and usual response (optimally controlled?).
- Co-morbidities affecting respiratory system (e.g. cardiac).

Examination

Look for abnormal findings, especially for complications of respiratory disease, such as pulmonary hypertension, right heart failure and steroid effects.

Functional

Simply asking the patient to lie flat and to climb stairs can provide very useful information.

Investigations

CXR

Request if history or clinical signs are suggestive of chest or cardiac disease.

ECG

Request for every patient >60 years and for younger patients if cardio-vascular or significant respiratory disease are present or suspected.

Spirometry

May provide useful information in the following circumstances.
- Evidence of significant respiratory disease.
- Equivocal clinical findings and uncertainty of diagnosis.
- Inability to ascertain exercise tolerance in patients with lower limb disability.
- To assess reversibility of pulmonary obstruction with beta-agonists or steroids.
- Prior to parenchymal lung resection.

FEV_1 <1 L increases the likelihood of postoperative respiratory complications and need for postoperative ventilation.

Cardiopulmonary exercise testing

This is a non-invasive objective method of evaluating both cardiac and pulmonary function. It may help to differentiate between cardiac and respiratory causes of dyspnoea. Variables measured include maximum oxygen consumption and anaerobic threshold.

Arterial blood gases

ABGs can identify chronic hypercapnic respiratory failure and are useful as a pre-operative baseline test in those with chronic respiratory disease.

Cigarette smoking

Effects
- Associated with COPD, cardiovascular disease, and lung malignancy.
- ↓ Mucociliary clearance.
- ↑ Airway reactivity → predisposes to coughing, bronchospasm, and laryngospasm.
- ↑ COHb → oxygen delivery ↓ (5–15% COHb in heavy smokers).
- Nicotine stimulates the sympathetic system → cardiac workload and coronary vascular resistance ↑.

Cessation
- It takes at least 8 weeks abstinence to see major benefits and reduced morbidity. In fact, cessation of <8 weeks may increase airway reactivity.
- Patients who are unable to stop smoking >8 weeks prior to surgery may still benefit from a 12–24 hour cessation, during which the nicotine and COHb levels normalize.

Further reading

British Thoracic Society (2001). BTS guidelines: guidelines on the selection of patients with lung cancer for surgery. *Thorax* **56**, 89–108.
British Thoracic Society: www.brit-thoracic.org.uk
NICE, Pre-operative tests. Available online at: www.nice.org.uk/pdf/CG3NICEguideline.pdf
Oxford Handbook of Respiratory Medicine, pp. 1–2.
Oxford Handbook of Anaesthesia, pp. 45–53.

Respiratory physiotherapy

Respiratory physiotherapy (PT) is indicated in specific acute situations to facilitate secretion clearance, reduce airflow obstruction and improve ventilation. This is achieved using a variety of airway clearance techniques.

Airway clearance techniques

Several airway clearance techniques (ACTs) are available and can be used alone or in combination according to the clinical situation.

- ACBT: the active cycle of breathing techniques is a group of breathing exercises used to aid/facilitate sputum expectoration. The three components are breathing control (BC), thoracic expansion exercises (TEE), and the forced expiration technique (FET).
- Gravity assisted postural drainage (PD) utilizes the anatomy of the main airways of the lung to allow specific positioning to drain a specific lung segment. Modified postural drainage uses the same principle but without the inclines being used.
- Manual techniques (MT) are percussion, vibration, and shakes performed manually by the PT on the patient.
- Autogenic drainage (AD): an airway clearance technique characterized by breathing control, with the emphasis on slow inspiration, then inspiratory pause followed by high expiratory flows whilst avoiding airway closure/collapse. The individual utilizes breathing at V_T, varying the depth within the inspiratory/expiratory reserve volumes according to the location of secretions, with the aim of mobilizing the secretions centrally from the peripheral airways. AD can be carried out independently or with assistance to apply overpressure.
- Positive expiratory pressure (PEP). Two devices are used in the UK: full face mask (Astra PEP) and a mouthpiece device (Pari PEP). The individual breathes in (no resistance) through the equipment using slightly larger than normal tidal volumes, and then exhales, generating a PEP of approximately 15 cmH$_2$O, as assessed by a (temporary) manometer in the circuit, due to a resistor in the circuit as prescribed by the PT. This is repeated five to eight times before performing an FET.
  - Oscillating PEP: a number of devices are available (flutter, cornet and acapella) which create oscillating PEP on the expiratory phase. They are used in a similar way to PEP devices.
- Intermittent positive pressure breathing (IPPB), also known as the Bird. IPPB is an adjunct to other ACTs. It is the application of volume-cycled pressure-limited support on inspiration via a mouthpiece or full face mask. It reduces the work of breathing, facilitating sputum clearance.
- Assisted cough techniques: these are manual techniques applied to the individual by the PT to augment cough strength during the coughing part of an appropriate airway clearance technique, when it is affected by neuromuscular weakness or mechanical disadvantage.
- CoughAssist (cough insufflation/exsufflation) applies positive and negative pressure to augment cough strength. It is applied via a full face mask or mouthpiece.

- Intermittent mandatory percussive ventilation (IMPV)/Percussionnaire: varying frequency, pressure, and inspiratory-to-expiratory ratio to maximize airway clearance.
- Suction: negative pressure via catheter inserted into lower airway via nasopharyngeal route, Guedel airway, tracheostomy, or mini-tracheostomy.
- Manual hyperinflation (MHI): used in patients with a tracheostomy unable to undertake conventional breathing exercises because of an acute deterioration. Using the 'bag', the physiotherapist can deliver normal V_T, MHI, inspiratory pauses, and fast expiratory releases to mimic huff/cough.
- Appropriate exercise: the use of graded exercises/mobilization can facilitate sputum clearance and lung volume recruitment.

Indications for physiotherapy

Sputum retention

Table 50.1 Interventions for sputum retention

	Pathophysiology	Possible PT intervention
Increased secretions or decreased mucociliary clearance	Increased sputum production, decreased mucociliary clearance, or altered rheological properties of sputum (such as in dehydration, poorly controlled diabetes, or CF)	ACBT, AD, PEP or oscillating PEP devices (i.e. ACTs), manual techniques, mobilization, postural drainage, IPPB
Ineffective cough, e.g. neuromuscular disease, decreased conscious level	Inspiratory volume limitation	ACTs, IPPB, NIV, IMPV, CoughAssist, suction (be clear whether for upper or lower airway secretion management)
	Limitation in expiratory force generation	ACTs, assisted cough techniques, CoughAssist, suction, cough lock

Sputum retention caused by bronchospasm should be managed medically, followed by PT if still appropriate

Patients with coexisting pain should have sufficient analgesia to allow full inspiration and cough. 'Wound support' or the use of a cough lock may be of assistance in some cases.

Tracheostomy patients
Consider tube patency, suction catheter size, and humidification/saline instillation. PT can add where routine suctioning by nursing staff has failed to manage the situation. ACTs, MHI, CoughAssist, and IPPB can be used.

Volume loss

Table 50.2 Interventions for volume loss

Pathophysiology	Possible PT intervention
Treatment strategies for decreased tidal volume (V_T) due to e.g. pain, fatigue, ↑ work of breathing (WOB), dynamic pulmonary hyperinflation	Consider mobilization, pain management, TEE, IPPB, MHI, relaxation, breathing control
Localized volume loss e.g. consolidation, collapse	ACTs, mobilization, positioning
Respiratory muscle weakness/fatigue	IPPB, NIV (Type II RF), positioning

Other causes of breathlessness

For conditions not amenable to physiotherapy treatment, the PT can advise regarding appropriate oxygen delivery, flow rates, humidification, and high flow devices.

Positioning can be used to ease breathlessness by managing active versus passive fixing and positions of ease, so that the work of breathing is reduced. V/Q matching can be utilized to optimize gas exchange, therefore easing breathlessness.

Contraindications and precautions

Contraindications to PT interventions should be discussed with the physiotherapist with respect to the individual patient. PT is not appropriate for breathlessness solely caused by the following.

- Pleural effusion/empyema.
- PE.
- Pneumonia (consolidated phase).
- Mass.
- Undrained pneumothorax/haemopneumothorax.
- Pulmonary oedema.
- Bronchospasm.
- Stridor.

On-call physiotherapy services

On-call physiotherapy services vary depending on local hospital policy, which will dictate whether the PT is on site or at home, with a specific time in which to attend a call-out.

The PT will ask specific questions to identify whether the problem is amenable to PT intervention and to identify specific contraindications to possible treatment.

Commonly asked questions

- Main symptom?
- What is the underlying pathology?
- Results of ABGs?
- FiO_2: delivery device, flow rate, humidification, and SaO_2.
- Results of recent CXR specifically regarding acute pathology and contraindications to the use of positive pressure if this is felt to be a possibility, e.g. bullous emphysema, undrained pneumothorax, some forms of lung cancer.
- CVS stability is important with regard to contraindications to some PT techniques.
- Fluid balance: hydration is an important component to sputum clearance.
- Pain management if appropriate: rib fractures, ICD, wound management. A patient may be pain free at rest, but may be unable to take a deep breath and/or cough.
- Is the patient able to follow commands?

Further reading

Harden B (2003). *An On-call Survival Guide: Emergency Physiotherapy*, pp. 79–118. Churchill Livingstone, Edinburgh.

Webber BA *et al.* (1998). Physiotherapy techniques. In Webber BA, Pryor JA, eds. *Physiotherapy for Respiratory and Cardiac Problems*, pp. 137–209. Churchill Livingstone, Edinburgh.

Hough A (1997). *Physiotherapy in Respiratory Care: A Problem-Solving Approach to Respiratory and Cardiac Management*. Stanley Thornes, Cheltenham.

Pleural aspiration

Pleural aspiration for diagnostic and therapeutic purposes is a commonly required procedure. Adequate attention must be paid to sterility and technique to prevent potential complications (bleeding, introduction of infection, and damage to the lung resulting in pneumothorax).

Aspiration may be required in three circumstances.
- Diagnostic evaluation of pleural effusion.
- Therapeutic relief of dyspnoea.
- Aspiration of pneumothorax.

Diagnostic aspiration

- Obtain written consent from the patient.
- Confirm the side of the effusion clinically and review a recent CXR to confirm.
- Position the patient sitting upright, leaning forward over a table (use pillow for comfort). Fold the patient's arms in front of them (moves the scapulae out of the way).
- Aspiration site.
  - Choose a rib space one or two spaces below where the chest becomes dull to percussion.
  - Approach may be posterior or lateral (mid-axillary line).
  - Avoid most posterior area (within about 3 cm of the erector spinae) as the intercostal artery often lies in the mid-intercostal space here.
- Prepare the skin (alcohol-based skin preparation) + aseptic technique.
- Infiltrate local anaesthetic.
  - Use 1% lidocaine 5–10 ml.
  - Initially raise a subcutaneous 'bleb'.
  - Advance while aspirating, aiming for just above the rib (avoids inferiorly placed neurovascular bundle).
  - Infiltrate tissues from skin through intercostal muscle to parietal pleura (may be painful).
  - You may feel a 'give' as you enter the pleural space.
- Aspirate fluid along anaesthetized tract (50 ml syringe, 21G needle).
- Note pleural fluid appearance.
- Send samples of fluid for:
  - biochemistry (protein, LDH, glucose).
  - microbiology (microscopy, culture ± AFBs).
  - cytology (if indicated).
  - pH (using blood gas machine).
- Post-procedure CXR is not routinely required.

Therapeutic aspiration

The same technique as for diagnostic aspiration is used (first seven steps above) initially. Then proceed as follows

- Essential to confirm that fluid is aspirated easily with the 21G needle used to infiltrate local anaesthetic. If fluid is not freely aspirated, image guidance (usually ultrasound) is required.
- Connect a three- way tap to a 50 ml syringe on one port and extension tubing on another.
- Insert a large-bore cannula (e.g. 16G) along the anaesthetized tract. You may feel a 'give' as you enter the pleural space as the parietal pleura is penetrated.
- Remove the needle to leave the plastic cannula within the chest. Therapeutic aspiration should not be conducted while the needle remains in the chest.
- Connect the cannula to the remaining port of the prepared three-way tap.
- Fluid can now be aspirated into the 50 ml syringe and expelled via the three-way tap and the extension tubing into a jug.
- Continue aspirating until resistance on aspiration OR significant cough or chest discomfort OR 1.5 L has been aspirated (possibly avoids risk of re-expansion pulmonary oedema).
- Note: removal of as little as 500 ml of fluid may result in substantial therapeutic benefit even in massive pleural effusion (as this decompresses hemithorax and improves respiratory mechanics).
- Clean and dress aspiration site.
- Repeat CXR after procedure (demonstrates degree of improvement or presence of pneumothorax).

Pneumothorax aspiration

The same technique (sterile preparation, skin infiltration) as above is used, with the following important differences.
- The patient is positioned lying at ~45°.
- The approach is anterior: second intercostal space in the mid-clavicular line.
- Pneumothorax is confirmed on aspirating air freely with the 21G local anaesthetic needle.
- Once the large-bore cannula has been placed, aspiration is conducted using the same 50 ml syringe–three-way tap assembly.
- Air is expelled via the three-way tap.
- Continue aspirating until resistance on aspiration OR significant cough or chest discomfort OR >2.5 L air aspirated (implies large air leak)—intercostal drainage is likely to be needed.
- Repeat CXR to document 'successful' aspiration.

Chest drain insertion

Although chest drains are used frequently, it should be remembered that there is a significant morbidity and even mortality associated with chest drain insertion. Complications increase with inexperienced operators, and the procedure must be undertaken or supervised by clinicians with experience in drain insertion. Chest drains are sometimes unnecessarily inserted (e.g. primary spontaneous pneumothorax), and careful thought should be given to the indication in each case.

Drain types

Trocar drain
- Stiff metal rod with a blunt end (trocar) sheathed in a plastic chest drain.
- Normally large size (24–32F).
- Inserted using blunt dissection technique (see later).
- Attempted insertion by exerting excessive pressure through the trocar on the chest wall can result in penetrating injury to the lung, heart, and great vessels, and may result in death.

Portex drain
- Similar plastic drain to above, but trocar is replaced with a flexible plastic introducer.
- Inserted using blunt dissection technique.

Seldinger drain
- Smaller flexible drains inserted using the Seldinger technique.
- Usually small (6–14F) but commercial kits are now available with 18F Seldinger drains.
- See section on insertion technique for further details.
- Although insertion technique is perceived to be 'easier' than for trocar or Portex drains, experience is required to prevent complications.

Radiologically inserted drain
- Generally smaller (<14F); inserted by Seldinger technique.
- Can be inserted using ultrasound or CT.
- Essential to request image guidance if doubt concerning radiological appearance, e.g. effusion versus consolidation/collapse or pneumothorax versus bulla.
- Essential to request image guidance if unable to aspirate fluid/air during insertion (see below).
- Particularly useful in multiloculated collections (especially empyema).

Indications for drain insertion

- Tension pneumothorax.
- Pneumothorax not responding to aspiration or likely to fail aspiration treatment.
- Complicated parapneumonic effusion/empyema.
- Malignant effusion (symptomatic relief ± chemical pleurodesis).
- Haemothorax.

Which size of drain to use?

Smaller drains (<14F) are adequate for most situations. Larger drains are advocated for the treatment of large air leaks in secondary pneumothorax, extensive surgical emphysema, and acute traumatic haemothorax.

There are no adequately powered clinical trials to guide optimal chest drain size selection. Observational studies suggest that smaller drains may be as effective and less painful than larger drains. If a smaller drain is used, regular flushes (30 ml sterile saline qds) will help keep the drain patent.

Cautions

- Lung adherent to chest wall (e.g. previous pleurodesis) is an absolute contraindication to chest drain insertion.
- Known coagulopathy should be corrected before drain insertion. Routine measurement of clotting/platelets is not required, but carefully consider the patient in front of you (e.g. known liver disease).
- Chest drains (or any medical procedure) must not be attempted unsupervised by those with inadequate experience and training.

Complications of chest drain insertion

- Pain.
- Infection (empyema results in up to 1%).
- Bleeding.
- Organ damage (e.g. liver, bowel in ~6%).
- 'Failure' (drain requires repositioning or reinserting).
- Vasovagal reactions are not uncommon.

Patients should give appropriate consent for the procedure and be informed of the complications.

Insertion technique

General preparation

- Obtain written consent.
- Confirm the side of the effusion clinically and on CXR.
- Premedication should be considered (e.g. midazolam 70–100 mcg/kg titrated to response (saturation monitoring required) OR diamorphine 2.5–5 mg (care in respiratory disease)).
- Ensure assistant available and drain bottle/tubing prepared.
- Choose drain insertion site:
  - Mid-axillary line, fourth to fifth intercostal space.
  - Aim for the 'triangle of safety' to avoid major vessels and nerves (an area posterior to pectoralis major, anterior to latisimus dorsi, and above the nipple line).
  - Avoid posterior approach where possible; patient will be unable to lie comfortably on their back.
- Three choices of patient position:
  - Lie patient at 45° with arm lifted behind head.
  - Lie patient flat in left or right lateral position.
  - Posterior approach (as for pleural aspiration); try to avoid in general.
- Sterile technique: don gloves and gown; prepare skin and drape area.
- Infiltrate with local anaesthetic as per pleural aspiration (1% lidocaine 10–20 ml may be required) and ensure pleural fluid (effusion) or air (pneumothorax) is aspirated easily using the 21G local anaesthetic needle.
- A longer needle (e.g. spinal needle) may be required in obese patients, but proceed cautiously.
- If fluid/air is not easily aspirated, abandon procedure and request image guidance.

Seldinger drain insertion

After steps above, proceed as follows.

- While waiting for local anaesthetic to take effect, open and prepare the Seldinger drain kit.
- Make a 5–7 m skin incision parallel to the ribs using the scalpel provided.
- Insert the introducer needle attached to the syringe. Carefully advance the needle while aspirating. The introducer needles are not sharp and should be advanced in a controlled manner. Advance until fluid/air is easily aspirated.
- Detach syringe and thread guidewire through introducer needle.
- From this point, one hand must always be holding the guidewire. Remove the introducer needle over the wire.
- Thread the dilator over the guidewire and insert 2–3 cm into the patient (no further). Withdraw the dilator over the wire.
- Thread the drain over the guidewire until the wire emerges from the distal end of the drain. Insert the drain smoothly into the pleural space whilst holding on to the guidewire. Insertion to 10–14 cm is usually adequate.

- Remove guidewire (+ plastic drain stiffener) and attach three-way tap.
- Insert a holding suture (a closing suture is not required) and secure with adhesive dressings (some well-designed dressings are commercially available).
- Connect to chest drain tubing and bottle. Ensure that:
  - drain is swinging
  - pleural fluid is draining (effusion) OR
  - drain is bubbling (pneumothorax).
- Ensure that patient is aware of good drain care (e.g. do not lift above waist height).
- Request CXR to confirm position.
- Document procedure in medical notes, including any complications/difficulties with drain insertion.

Blunt dissection insertion (trocar/Portex)

After general preparation:
- Make a 7–10 mm skin incision parallel to the ribs using a scalpel.
- Place a horizontal mattress suture across the wound using strong suture material (e.g. 1 silk). Purse string sutures are no longer advised as they leave larger scars and are painful.
- Create a tract for drain entry by blunt dissection using blunt forceps (e.g. Spencer–Wells) as follows.
  - Insert forceps (closed) into the incision and exert gentle pressure on the underlying tissue.
  - Open the forceps (separates underlying tissue).
  - Withdraw forceps completely while open.
  - Reinsert closed forceps and repeat steps above.
- The forceps should never be withdrawn in the closed position. This risks avulsion and damage to tissues.
- A 'give' will be felt on penetrating the parietal pleura. This may take some time, but attempting to rush blunt dissection can result in injury.
- Pass the drain (+ trocar/plastic stiffener) into the pleural space through the tract created. The drain should pass easily with minimal pressure.
- If there is resistance to passing the drain, DO NOT exert firmer pressure (risks penetrating injury). Instead, repeat blunt dissection to re-create a tract and then attempt to re-pass the drain.
- Once the drain is in place, insert a holding suture.
- Continue management as per Seldinger drain insertion.

Further reading

Laws D et al. (2003). BTS guidelines for insertion of a chest drain. *Thorax*, **58** (Suppl 2), ii53–4.

Part 6

Investigations

Arterial blood gases

Arterial blood gas (ABGs) analysis forms the cornerstone of emergency respiratory investigation. In many situations values obtained dictate management strategy and facilitate decision-making. It is an uncomfortable procedure for the patients and if repeated ABGs are required, consider whether less invasive measures, such as respiratory rate, pulse oximetry or capillary blood gas measurements could be used.

> Prior to every ABG decide how the result will
> CHANGE MANAGEMENT

Principles

Technique and analysis

- Radial artery most commonly punctured. Alternative sites include femoral, ulnar or brachial arteries.
- Capillary ear lobe samples can be used but can be difficult to obtain in an emergency setting.
- Introduction of a small superficial bleb of 1% lidocaine has been shown to significantly reduce levels of patient discomfort.
- If frequent gases are needed (e.g. commencing non-invasive ventilation) consider placement of an arterial line (see below).
- Transport on ice is unnecessary if time to analysis is less than 10 minutes.
- Pre-analytical errors should be kept to minimum – see below.
- Analysis after change in therapy depends upon alveolar ventilation. 5 minutes is sufficient in most cases, however in obstructive airways disease steady state change may take up to 30 minutes.
- **Always record** the current FiO_2 and level of ventilatory support (as relevant).

The analyzer

- **Beware** some values are measured (PaO_2, $PaCO_2$, pH) and others are 'calculated' (HCO_3, TCO, Base excess, and often SaO_2 – unless co-oximeter–see pulse oximetry chapter). Calculated values are obtained from standardized equations that may not be appropriate or indeed accurate in critically ill patients.
- It is not uncommon for a busy machine to become decalibrated (e.g. over a bank holiday weekend) and therefore interpret unexpected results with caution.

ABG analytical errors

- **Too much heparin:** Liquid heparin must be expelled prior to sample collection (a small amount will always remain). The PaO_2 and $PaCO_2$ of heparin is virtually the same as ambient air and therefore heparin dilution will move the PaO_2 towards atmospheric values and (because it is acidic) lower the pH. Dry heparin syringes reduce this risk and allow for more accurate electrolyte calculation.
- **Exposed to air:** Sample will tend toward ambient room values. $PaCO_2$ reduced, pH increased.
- **Slow analysis:** aside from exposure to air, blood continues to metabolize and hence the PaO_2 decreases, $PaCO_2$ increases and pH falls.
- **? Venous:** is often seen scrawled next to ABG printouts. Pulsatile flow may be poor in the critically ill patient. Compare SaO_2 with pulse oximeter – usually fairly good correlation, however, if there is still clinically significant doubt analyse a venous sample.
- **Temperature correction?** Most blood gas analyzers maintain the electrode at 37°C. If the patient is relatively hypothermic, the electrode will heat the sample and reduce the Hb affinity, raising the PaO_2 (the reverse is also true). Most analyzers incorporate equations to adjust for this effect (and hence change all calculated values). Changes in acid base status may reflect in vivo homeostasis and therefore should be interpreted according to unadjusted values.

When to consider an Arterial Line in respiratory emergencies

- In the **critically ill patient** who is likely to need close blood pressure monitoring (e.g. in setting of inotrope use, haemodynamically unstable).
- Those likely to **need multiple ABGs**. Patients on non-invasive ventilation often fall into this group however consider other variables that can be used to assess progress; transcutaneous CO_2 monitoring has been shown to be useful.

When placing a line consider

- Remember Allen's Test prior to insertion (testing patency of ulnar and radial arterial flow) – demonstrated at web-link below.
- Ensure every sample taken has implications for management.
- Venesection of patient if multiple samples taken (including wastage for clearing line) – watch for falling Hb.
- Remove at first opportunity – infectious risk lower than venous access but remains source of sepsis.

Technique is demonstrated in video at link http://content.nejm.org/cgi/video/354/15/e13/

Simple questions for ABG interpretation

It is important to consider the following questions to optimize interpretation. They can be approached in any order:

1) Is this sample correctly analyzed?
Reduce analytical errors -See previous page.

2) What does the ABG tell you about oxygen delivery?
See oxygen chapter for more details but key is SaO_2, PaO_2 and Hb (if measured). Patients are often on high FiO_2 and therefore it is important to always record and consider the FiO_2. E.g. PaO_2 14 on FiO_2 0.6 (60 %) is not good!

> **Quick Check**
>
> Is the PaO_2 as high as expected?
> If the $PaCO_2$ is normal, then the
>
> PaO_2 (kPa) approximately = FiO_2 (%) x 0.75 e.g. as above 60 x 0.75
>
> $\qquad\qquad\qquad\qquad\qquad = 45$ Kpa

In addition to conditions that cause V/Q mismatch or shunting, a low PaO_2 may also arise due to hypoventilation – therefore one needs to calculate the A-a gradient (see below).

3) What is the $PaCO_2$?
$PaCO_2$ will give clues regarding ventilation – less than 4.0 kPa suggests hyperventilation, greater than 6.0 kPa suggesting hypoventilation. It is important to remember that 'hypoventilation' may reflect an imbalance between load and capacity and not simply a low RR.

4) What is the pH?
If an acid base disturbance is present, determine the nature of the disturbance (see below). Beware compensation and look at base excess and HCO_3, significant disturbances may underlie a near normal pH.

5) What other information can help?
Look at all the information – view and record Mg, Lactate and COHb (is the patient still smoking?).

The Alveolar to arterial gradient made simple

The A–a gradient is a measure of how efficiently the respiratory exchange surface is functioning. If the alveolus is packed with CO_2 then there is less O_2 to exchange and this is reflected in the PaO_2. Calculating the A–a gradient allows determination of oxygen exchange with respect to CO_2 and FiO_2.

Example: In a drowsy patient with an elevated $PaCO_2$ and low PaO_2 the A–a gradient helps determine if the poor saturations can be purely attributed to hypoventilation or if there is an underlying abnormality of oxygen exchange. e.g. pulmonary embolus.

How is it calculated?

$$\text{A–a gradient} = \text{Alveolar } PO_2 - (PaO_2 + PaCO_2/R)$$

The alveolar oxygen needs to be adjusted according to the FiO_2, atmospheric pressure (100kPa) and water vapour pressure (7 kPa) as follows:

FiO_2 Air, $21/100 \times (100 - 7)$ approx. 20 kPa

FiO_2 24%, $24/100 \times (100 - 7)$ approx. 23 kPa

FiO_2 35%, $35/100 \times (100 - 7)$ approx. 33 kPa

Respiratory Quotient (R) for purposes of on-call calculation = 0.8 (easier to multiply by 1.2).

EXAMPLE

e.g. If breathing air (FiO_2 = 21 kPa), PaO_2 = 13kPa and $PaCO_2$ = 4.8 kPa

Then the alveolar oxygen is 20

A–a gradient = $20 - (13+4.8/0.8) = 1$

What is Normal?
It is normal to have a small A–a gradient as, even in the normal lung, there is not perfect ventilation to perfusion matching. Values increase with age and are usually 1–2, increasing to 2–3 in the elderly.

Acid Base balance, pH and Respiratory Emergencies

Key to acid base analysis is remembering that homeostasis is centered on maintaining near normal pH; compensations are made to correct towards normal pH.

Larger texts describe in detail the nature of acid base abnormalities and compensatory mechanisms (see OHRM p722) however the most commonly encountered derangements in respiratory emergencies are:

Respiratory Acidosis
$1°$ *disturbance*: inadequate ventilation (best thought of as an imbalance between load on the system vs. capacity) leading to elevated CO_2 and hence acidosis, e.g. neuromuscular respiratory failure.

Compensatory mechanism: retain HCO_3. Note some HCO_3 elevation occurs by virtue of acute buffering (haemoglobin and proteins). It is very unusual for full compensation to occur – therefore the primary disturbance can usually be deduced (although not in mixed pattern). Compensation occurs over a number of hours/days and hence pH and HCO_3 provide clues to the chronicity of a respiratory acidosis.

Respiratory Alkalosis

1° disturbance: 'over' ventilation with low $PaCO_2$. E.g. hyperventilation. Can also occur in pathological conditions e.g. pulmonary embolism and asthma.

Compensatory mechanism: waste HCO_3 leading to negative base excess. This can give clues to 'chronicity' of dyspnoea.

Metabolic Acidosis

1° disturbance: metabolic acid excess. In emergencies think about lactate, renal function, glucose, drugs, toxins and alcohol. If still unclear then determine anion gap (normal range = 8–16 mmol/L).

$$\text{Anion gap} = [K^+] + [Na^+] - [Cl^-] - [HCO_3]$$

Tissue hypoxia leads to anaerobic metabolism and hence lactate prodution.

> Large doses of salbutamol can give rise to lactic acidosis.

Metabolic acidosis and ↑ anion gap

Due to increased production of fixed/organic acids:
- Lactic acidosis – shock, infection, hypoxia.
- Renal failure.
- DKA (and ketone production in alcohol excess).
- Drugs/toxins (salicylates, biguanides, ethylene glycol, methanol).

Metabolic acidosis and normal anion gap

Due to loss of bicarbonate or ingestion of H+ ions:
- Renal tubular acidosis.
- Diarrhoea.
- Drugs (acetazolamide).
- Addison's disease.
- Pancreatic fistula.

Compensatory mechanism: increased ventilatory drive with reduced $PaCO_2$ – occurs acutely. May explain why acidotic patient appears breathless and underpins why respiratory rate is such a sensitive marker for detecting the acutely unwell medical patient (as part of emergency warning scores).

Tips for acid base interpretation

- A falling pH in a patient with respiratory failure may occur secondary to a change in the metabolic component. e.g. secondary to lactic acidaemia. **Beware attributing falling pH to ventilatory deterioration.**
- pH is key to acute management decisions in ventilatory failure – see NIV chapter. In decompensation an approximate correction can be made for the pH to estimate where the 'chronic' $PaCO_2$ normally 'sits':

For every increase in $PaCO_2$ of 2.6 kPa above normal the pH falls by 0.1.

For every decrease of $PaCO_2$ of 1.3 kPa below normal the pH rises by 0.1. Although this relationship is not entirely linear it can be used as a useful trick.

e.g. *in decompensated acute on chronic respiratory failure if the pH is 7.25 and the $PaCO_2$ 9.0, (providing the pH disturbance is predominantly respiratory), one would expect a $PaCO_2$ at 'compensation' (i.e. above 7.35) to be 9.0–2.6 –6.4.*

Other Methods for assessing CO_2

Transcutaneous CO_2

Recent evidence suggests that $PaCO_2$ can be monitored using transcutaneous skin monitors. These have been previously used successfully in sleep laboratories but can be used to manage patients on NIV. Limitations include cost, risk of thermal skin burns and skill requirement (poor care can lead to sensor damage).

End tidal CO_2

On call general physicians will most commonly encounter this technique when it is employed to monitor intubated patients. The technique utilizes the principles of absorption spectroscopy to measure CO_2 in expired gas. It is most useful for detecting ET tube displacement (gastric trace obtained) and when transferring critically ill patients.

Pulse oximetry

Pulse oximetry

When employed correctly, pulse oximetry is a rapid non-invasive method of assessing one of the key components of tissue oxygen delivery: the oxygen saturation of haemoglobin (SaO_2).

Principles and application

- Based on the laws of light absorbance and optical density (Lambert's law and Beer's law), i.e. the principle that deoxygenated and oxygenated hemoglobin absorb light at different wavelengths.
- The accuracy of modern pulse oximeters is ± 2%, although they are less accurate in lower saturation ranges. When inaccuracies occur saturation is usually underestimated. However, this underlines the need for **caution when reliance is placed on an absolute figure**, i.e. as a screening tool to avoid arterial blood gas sampling.
- A number of factors can affect accuracy and cause problems (see box opposite).

Pulse oximetry versus co-oximetry

- Pulse oximeters measure oxygen saturation SpO_2. This differs from the arterial saturation value (SaO_2) obtained in blood gas analysers with a co-oximeter. In the latter, a larger number of wavelengths allow the measurement of other haemoglobin types:

$$SaO_2 = HbO_2/(HbO_2 + Hb + COHb + metHB) \times 100\%.$$

In clinical practice the terms SpO_2 and SaO_2 are often used interchangeably. In the majority of circumstances this is of no consequence However, it is important to understand that there is a difference.

- ❶ **Beware** Some analysers are not co-oximeters and simply determine SaO_2 for wavelengths as per a finger probe.
- Co-oximetry is necessary in the management of carbon monoxide (CO) poisoning. COHb has similar absorbance and therefore mimics the presence of oxyhaemoglobin. This leads to falsely elevated SaO_2 readings on a standard saturation monitor.
- Smoking can also increase CO levels (often used in smoking cessation clinics as a tool to assess compliance) and can lead to SaO_2 inaccuracy (falsely elevated).

Other uses

Overnight oximetry can be used to assess nocturnal desaturation in sleep disorder breathing.

Problems with pulse oximetry

Common
- Signal quality: often due to probe application. Can try tape to secure probe or earlobe device.
- Tissue perfusion, e.g. hypotension.
- Body temperature.
- Penumbra: light shunting around the finger gives falsely low SaO_2.

Uncommon
- Nail varnish: effect depends upon colour. Green and blue reduce SaO_2 reading, but red usually has no effect. Aim to remove all varnish to obtain optimum reading.
- Anaemia (Hb <5).

Rare (low SaO_2 with no apparent explanation)
- Dyshaemoglobinaemia (see co-oximeter entry above), e.g. methaemoglobinaemia. The wavelength light absorption leads SaO_2 towards 85%.
- Intravascular dyes.

For more details see Hurford WE, Kratz A (2004). Case records of the Massachusetts General Hospital. Weekly clinicopathological exercises. Case 23–2004. A 50-year-old woman with low oxygen saturation. *N Engl J Med* **351**, 380–7.

Peak flow

Peak flow

Peak flow is defined as the greatest expiratory flow achieved from a maximally forced expiratory effort when starting from a position of full inspiration.

Principles and application

- Measurement should be performed as best of three with standardized meter (EU scale). There is no need to return the measuring plunger to zero following each attempt.
- Result is effort dependent.
- Circadian changes are well recognized: peaks at 16.00, nadir at 04.00.
- Guidelines suggest cut-off values to determine severity of acute asthma and dictate treatment. However, trends and response to treatment are more useful than absolute values. For reference range see Fig. 55.1.
- PEFR is affected by changes in large airway calibre and therefore is of limited value in the assessment of COPD.
- PEFR has no value in discriminating restrictive from obstructive disease: restrictive conditions will limit ability to generate high PEFR.

When NOT to use PEFR

- PEFR measurement should not be attempted in suspected life-threatening acute asthma It is unlikely to change management and may cause cardiovascular collapse (due to intra-pleural pressure changes).
- As a substitute for FVC measurement in the management of neuromuscular respiratory failure.
- When deciding if a patient has an obstructive or restrictive pulmonary disorder. Not a substitute for spirometry.
- As the only decision variable for discharging asthmatics.

Cough peak flow

Peak expiratory flow during cough (cough PEF) is a useful adjunct in the assessment of patients with suspected neuromuscular respiratory failure. Values below 150 L/min suggest poor airway clearance and should prompt consideration of further investigation and intervention to ensure adequate management.

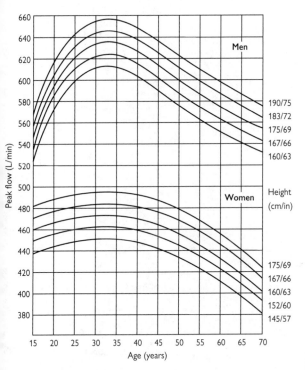

Fig. 55.1 Peak flow reference ranges. (With kind permission from *The Oxford Handbook of Respiratory Medicine*.)

Spirometry

Spirometry

When performed correctly, spirometry is a valuable tool which helps to classify a respiratory disorder. It is rarely indicated in the acute emergency setting; although is of significant importance in the management of patients with neuromuscular respiratory failure (FVC monitoring).

Principles

- Modern hand-held electronic devices allow simple analysis.
- Effort and technique dependent. The patient breathes at tidal volume, then inhales slowly to total lung capacity (TLC), and then exhales as hard and fast as possible to residual volume (RV). Encouragement should be given to ensure maximum force and continuation. It is important to use a spirometer with a volume–time trace to ensure that the true FVC obtained.
- Repeatability is the key to ensuring that adequate patient effort has been obtained.
- Many devices enable calculation of a predicted value (for age, sex and height). If they do not, good calculators are available at: http://www.cdc.gov/niosh/topics/spirometry/RefCalculator.html
- When interpreting values, 'normal' is usually taken to include values >80% of the predicted value. However, it is perhaps more useful to consider predicted values in terms of a range around the population mean $\pm$ 1.64 $\times$ standard deviation.
- It is important to consider the population data you are using. There are no accurate population data for people aged >85 years.
- Do not confuse the results for the FEV_1/FVC ratio (FER) and the percentage predicted figure with that ratio sometimes given on electronic printouts. Use the actual percentage (in bold below). For example,

    FEV_1 = 1.94, FVC = 2.60, age 50 years, height 1.60 m

    FEV_1/FVC = 74%

    Percentage predicted 90%

Spirometry application
- Most commonly used to distinguish restrictive from obstructive disorders. FEV_1/FVC <0.7 is suggestive of the latter (see Table 56.1).
- In restrictive disorders the ratio is usually preserved due to fall in FVC. ❶ Beware. Not all falls in FVC are due to restrictive disease. FVC also falls if RV is elevated (due to air trapping) (see Fig 56.1).
- Percentage predicted values for FEV_1 help to classify severity of disease in COPD and guide treatment (📖 Chapter 21). FEV_1 does not change significantly during exacerbations and is of limited value in monitoring.
- FVC monitoring in neuromuscular respiratory failure: if the diaphragm is paralysed then on lying flat the abdominal contents limit inspiration. Early failure may be detected by supine drop in FVC:
- 10–20 % is suspicious; >20% is definitely abnormal and suggests significance, usually bilateral paralysis. (Note: Drops by 5% in normal subjects.) Do not substitute PEFR for FVC in this condition.

For more details see OHRM, pp. 708–11.

Further pulmonary function tests

A number of other pulmonary function tests are widely available and used in respiratory medicine (e.g. formal lung function tests/body plethymography, transfer factor analysis). However, in the **emergency setting** it is probably more important to ask the following questions.
- Will the investigation I am requesting change management acutely?
- Can the patient safely undergo the investigation and perform sufficiently to achieve a meaningful result?
- Do I know what the 'normal' values should be and how a certain result is interpreted?

For example, in the setting of suspected acute pulmonary haemorrhage requesting transfer factor analysis. Visit the pulmonary function technicians and discuss what is feasible and sensible. Novel techniques may be available (such as using trans-diaphragmatic pressure recordings), but again ask local specialist/technicians for advice.

The Empey index

The Empey index is a method of predicting whether a patient has upper airways obstruction:

Empey index = FEV_1/PEFR.

In the presence of upper airways obstruction PEFR is reduced disproportionately to FEV_1. A figure >10 supports the presence of upper airways obstruction. The index has been used at the bedside to support a diagnosis of tracheal stenosis:[1]

---

1 France JE, Thomas MJ (2004). Clinical use of the Empey index in the emergency department. *Emerg Med J* **21**, 642–3.

Table 56.1 Pattern of lung volume change found in obstructive and restrictive lung disease

Derivative	Obstructive	Restrictive
FEV₁ (% predicted)	↓↓	↓
VC (% predicted)	↓ or →	↓
FEV₁/VC ratio	↓	→ or ↑ (increased recoil)
TLC (% predicted)	↑ or →	↓
RV (% predicted)	↑	↓
FRC (% predicted)	↑	↓
RV/TLC ratio	↑ (gas trapping)	↓

With kind permission from *The Oxford Handbook of Respiratory Medicine.*

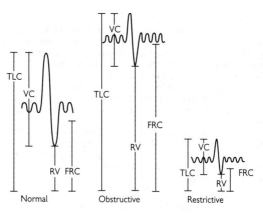

Fig. 56.1 Lung volumes in normal, obstructive, and restrictive lung conditions: TLC, total lung capacity; VC, vital capacity; RV, residual volume; FRC, functional residual capacity; FEV₁, forced expiratory volume in 1 second. (With kind permission from *The Oxford Handbook of Respiratory Medicine.*)

Bronchoscopy

Bronchoscopy

Bronchoscopy involves the passage of a fibreoptic bronchoscope, through the upper airways, past the vocal cords, and into the lungs. The upper and lower airways can be examined, samples can be taken for diagnosis and treatment can be carried out if necessary. There are only a few indications for urgent bronchoscopy, which are discussed below. The opinion of a respiratory physician should be sought.

Indications for urgent bronchoscopy

Foreign body
Usually associated with a clear history of aspiration. CXR may show the foreign body if radio-opaque, or may show an area of atelectasis or hyperinflation on a post-expiration film. The most common site for aspiration is the right lower lobe. Bronchoscopy is only required urgently if there is respiratory distress.

Thoracic trauma
Bronchoscopy might be required to exclude serious airway injury such as tracheobronchial fracture. May also reveal aspirated foreign bodies or be useful therapeutically for removal of mucous plugs.

Massive haemoptysis
Occasionally indicated in massive haemoptysis. Can be a useful test to localize the site of bleeding. If bleeding is localized to a distal bronchus attempt to tamponade by wedging the bronchoscope into the bronchus. Iced saline can be irrigated or use 1 ml aliquots of 1:10 000 adrenaline onto the bleeding point to arrest the bleeding. If available, attempt to coagulate the bleeding point. Uncontrollable bleeding ideally requires a rigid bronchoscope, usually only done by thoracic surgeons.

Causes include neoplasm, tuberculous cavities, aspergillomas, pulmonary alveolar haemorrhage syndromes, bronchiectasis, and cystic fibrosis. Death occurs secondary to asphyxiation not exsanguination. If there is massive bleeding turn patient onto the side of the bleeding to protect the other lung. Consider intubation with double lumen tube (Chapter 6).

Usual indications for bronchoscopy

- Suspected lung cancer, for staging and histology or cytology.
- Suspected mycobacterial disease, where the patient is unable to produce sputum.
- In the immunocompromised patient with fever/hypoxia/pulmonary infiltrates (Chapter 13).
- Diffuse interstitial lung disease: transbronchial biopsy for histology. Often positive in sarcoidosis but less helpful in other conditions.
- For therapeutic intervention, e.g. stenting, diathermy.

Contraindications

- Unstable cardiovascular state, including arrhythmias.
- Severe hypoxaemia that is likely to worsen during the procedure.
- Uncooperative patient.
- Rigid bronchoscopy is contraindicated in those with severe ankylosing spondylitis of the neck or in the presence of an unstable cervical spine.

Preparation pre-bronchoscopy
- Full history including allergies and previous response to anaesthetic.
- Examination or cardiovascular and respiratory systems.
- CXR.
- Clotting screen and platelet count if intervention procedures likely or if on anticoagulants or concerns re clotting status (e.g. liver metastases, uraemia).
- Fast for 4 hours pre-procedure.
- Consent.

Other considerations pre-bronchoscopy
- If the patient is asthmatic, consider pre-bronchoscopy nebulizer of short-acting beta-agonist.
- Because of the requirement to be nil by mouth pre-bronchoscopy, consideration must be given to diabetics' medication.
- ❶ Those at risk of endocarditis should receive appropriate prophylaxis pre-bronchoscopy, usually amoxicillin 3 g po 1 hour before.

Complications
Mortality and morbidity are low with bronchoscopy. However, complications can arise related to the use of sedation, topical anaesthetics, or the procedure itself.

Complications from sedation include respiratory depression, syncope and hypotension. Rarely, topical anaesthetics may cause laryngospasm or bronchospasm. Cardiac arrhythmias occur in ~0.5%. Haemorrhage associated with biopsy is one of the major complications and should be treated as discussed earlier in the chapter. Death related to bronchoscopy is extremely rare, occurring in <0.04%.

Patient post-bronchoscopy
Up to one-third of patients will develop fever after bronchoscopy and lavage (induced by cytokine release from alveolar macrophages). This will settle without antibiotics, although antipyretics such as paracetamol can be used.

In patients who have undergone interventional bronchoscopy such as diathermy or stenting, fever post-bronchoscopy should be treated with antibiotics (e.g. Augmentin® or doxycycline) as it is more likely to be due to infection.

Major complications include the following.
- **Post-biopsy haemorrhage:** if small volume then likely to settle. Consider admission for observation, particularly if significant volumes. 📖 Chapter 6 for management.
- **Pneumothorax**: occurs in ~10% after transbronchial lung biopsy. Consider in those presenting with chest pain and/or increased shortness of breath. Perform CXR and treat as per secondary pneumothorax.

Radiology

Introduction

Because of its portable nature and rapid interpretation, the PA chest X-ray (CXR) (Fig. 58.1) remains the most useful radiological investigation for the patient with acute respiratory symptoms. Accurate assessment of the CXR is based on a combination of pattern recognition and a logical approach to ensure that important features on the film are not missed or misinterpreted. The experienced physician will use the CXR to assess not only the lungs, but also the trachea, mediastinum, hila, pleura, bones, and chest wall.

In this chapter we describe the important CXR patterns for the most common respiratory emergencies. If another imaging modality is needed to confirm the diagnosis, the investigation of choice will be described. There are numerous pitfalls that can cause important pathologies to be missed on the CXR, and others that cause over-diagnosis. The most frequent of these pitfalls are described, together with indications for urgent input from the on-call radiologist.

Infection

The CXR appearances of infection are extremely varied. A bacterial infection causing community-acquired pneumonia (CAP) may be seen as a solitary focus of consolidation, whereas PCP in the immunocompromised patient typically causes a bilateral peri-hilar infiltrate. Whilst familiarity with the features of CAP on CXR will enable prompt treatment to be started, the physician must also recognize complications of infection, such as a lung abscess or cavitation. The indicative signs for an atypical, viral, or fungal infection must also be known.

CXR features of bacterial CAP (Fig. 58.2)

- Consolidation (dense shadowing that obscures blood vessels), often with air bronchograms (visible airways within the shadowing).
- Lower lobes most commonly affected.
- Pleural effusion is common, but lymphadenopathy is uncommon.
- A more diffuse interstitial and infiltrative pattern can be seen without focal consolidation.
- Consolidation can appear as a discrete focal mass, mimicking or possibly obscuring an underlying malignancy. ❶ A repeat CXR 6 weeks after treatment is advised to exclude a lung cancer.
- Multifocal consolidation can be seen, particularly in streptococcal infection.

Other CXR features: consider atypical infection

- Cavitation (round lucency, often multifocal): seen especially with *Staphylococcus aureus infection*. Pneumothorax (PTX) can be a complication.
- Differential of cavitation on the CXR.
  - Infection: predominantly staphylococcus, but also anaerobes and fungal.

- Tuberculosis (TB).
- Carcinoma.
- Granulomatous vasculitis.
- Rheumatoid nodules.
- Upper lobe predilection: seen especially with *Klebsiella* and TB.
- Lower lobe predilection: seen especially with *Legionella*.

CXR features of viral pneumonia
- Bilateral diffuse infiltrate as opposed to focal consolidation.
- Multiple nodules,1–5 mm in diameter.
- Calcification of nodules implies prior, not active, infection (especially varicella).
- Effusions and hilar lymphadenopathy are not typically present.
- Bacterial infection can complicate viral pneumonia.

CXR features of fungal infection
Variable findings, but there is generally a diffuse infiltrative or nodular appearance. Some fungal infections have specific CXR features.
- Aspergilloma or mycetoma: usually an apical cavity containing a fungal ball of soft tissue density. Surrounding crescent of air visible (halo sign). A complication of cavitatory TB.
- Bronchopulmonary aspergillosis: CXR shows central bronchiectasis (airway dilatation). Mucoid impaction within these dilated airways gives a 'finger in glove' appearance.
- PCP: bilateral peri-hilar opacity. Occasionally small cysts may be seen. CXR normal in 10%. PTX a common complication. PCP should be considered in at-risk patients presenting with pneumothorax.

Tuberculosis
TB has perhaps the most variable appearance on CXR of any infection, sometimes complicated by prior surgical treatment. Certain CXR features should alert the clinician to the possibility of tuberculous disease, although comparison with old films is often necessary to assess whether CXR abnormalities are longstanding (Fig. 58.3).

CXR features suggestive of TB
- Upper lobe consolidation.
- Hilar or paratracheal lymph node enlargement. Main differential is sarcoid (Fig. 58.4).
- Cavitation (hallmark of reactivation), possibly with mycetoma.
- Multiple nodules 2–3 mm in size are characteristic of miliary TB (diffuse haematogenous spread).

Role of ultrasound and CT

An ultrasound scan (US) should be performed if an effusion or empyema is suspected and the CXR is not diagnostic. If a lung abscess is suspected, CT is highly sensitive and specific. Some lung abscesses are amenable to percutaneous drainage under CT guidance.

High-resolution CT scanning (HRCT) is the investigation of choice when fungal infection is suspected, especially for patients who are immuno-compromised. Some organisms, particularly PCP and invasive aspergillosis, have characteristic appearances on HRCT, and this investigation can be diagnostic.

Pneumothorax

PTX is air in the pleural space, with consequent collapse of adjacent lung. The key CXR features are listed below. If a tension PTX is suspected and there are signs of imminent cardiovascular compromise, treatment should be undertaken *before* the CXR is performed.

CXR features (Figs 58.5 and 58.6)

- Abnormal lucency (blackness) within a hemithorax.
- Shift of trachea/mediastinum away from side of PTX (consider carefully whether tension PTX exists).
- A thin white line representing the visceral pleura may be seen, separating collapsed lung from air in the pleural space.
- Absence of vascular markings (although this is normal in the lung periphery).
- A ruptured pleural bleb may be seen in spontaneous PTX.
- Ipsilateral blunting of the costophrenic angle.
- Abnormal prominence and depth of the ipsilateral costophrenic angle (deep sulcus sign). Seen if patient has been imaged supine (e.g. ventilated patient on ITU).
- Medial diaphragm clearly outlined through cardiac silhouette or abnormal sharpness of a cardiac border, again usually seen in a supine patient with air lying anteriorly in the thorax.

Common pitfalls

- A rotated film can cause apparent lucency of one hemithorax (common when a portable CXR has been taken).
- Mistaking overlying clothing or even hair for the pleural edge.
- Bullae (in context of COPD) can mimic PTX as both cause abnormal lucency.

Further investigations

- Lateral decubitus or expiratory frontal CXR can reveal a small PTX not readily visible on the erect CXR.
- CT thorax is occasionally indicated in the context of gross bullous changes or presence of extensive surgical emphysema, making the CXR difficult to interpret.

Pulmonary embolism

Although there are no specific diagnostic CXR features, it should still be performed to exclude other pathologies.

Non-specific CXR features (often normal)

- Small pleural effusion (usually exudate).
- Atelectasis (a focal area of collapse, usually linear or wedge-shaped).
- Decreased vascularity (causing increased lucency of a lobe or hemithorax).
- Prominence of a pulmonary artery.
- Raised hemidiaphragm.

Further investigations

CT pulmonary angiogram (CTPA)

- The investigation of choice with a sensitivity >95%.
- Requires 100 ml of IV contrast through a large-bore peripheral cannula.
- Contraindicated if the patient has renal failure, severe asthma, or a history of allergy to iodine.
- Acute emboli seen as low-attenuation filling defects in pulmonary vasculature.
- CTPA has the advantage of demonstrating other causes for respiratory symptoms in the absence of PE.

Isotope lung scan (ventilation/perfusion or V/Q scan)

- Ventilation and lung perfusion are studied by measuring the radioactivity of inhaled and injected particles. A perfusion defect in an area of normal ventilation is indicative of thrombus.
- Useful as a first-line investigation in patients with a normal CXR and no cardiac or pulmonary disease.
- Most commonly, only Q scan performed.
- Abnormal CXR often gives an indeterminate scan.
- CTPA preferred in most centres, although Q scan useful if CTPA is contraindicated and CXR is normal.

Out-of-hours availability

Many hospitals do not provide on-call nuclear medicine studies. CTPA can be delayed until normal working hours if there is no contraindication to anticoagulation in the interim.

Pleural effusion and empyema

Pleural effusion

Most effusions are easily seen on CXR and do not require further imaging.

CXR features (Figs. 58.7 and 58.8)

- Basal opacity obscuring the hemidiaphragms.
- Meniscus curving upwards at the medial/lateral edges on the frontal view.
- Large effusions cause the mediastinum to be pushed *away* (cf. lobar collapse).
- Small effusions: only feature may be 'blunting' of the costophrenic angle.

Pitfalls

- Up to 200 ml of fluid can collect in the posterior recess and may not be seen on the PA CXR (a lateral CXR or US may be helpful).
- Fluid can also collect in the subpulmonic space, which is above the hemidiaphragm and inferior to the lung. The appearance is of an elevated hemidiaphragm, but with an abnormal lateral peak.

Empyema

This is infected pleural fluid and requires aspiration or drainage. The CXR cannot confirm or exclude whether pleural fluid is infected. US is useful for guiding percutaneous aspiration or chest drain insertion. This is especially true if the collection is small and/or loculated. If a patient with a chest infection remains septic despite treatment, a CT of the thorax will identify if an empyema or abscess is present.

CT features of empyema

- Low-attenuation collection between lung and the chest wall/mediastinum/diaphragm.
- Visceral and parietal pleura are separated.
- Pleura is thickened and shows avid enhancement with IV contrast.
- Foci of gas within the empyema (prior to pleural instrumentation) are suggestive of development of a bronchopleural fistula.

Pulmonary oedema and ARDS

There are many non-cardiac causes of pulmonary oedema and ARDS. These two pathologies are considered together as many of the CXR features overlap (the heart size and clinical presentation usually allow differentiation of the two). ARDS is common in ITU patients as a result of sepsis, aspiration, or DIC. Inhalation of smoke or overdose from opiate abuse are other causes. CXR features can lag behind the clinical status by 12–24 hours.

CXR features (Fig. 58.9)

- Prominence of upper lobe blood vessels ('upper lobe diversion').
- Peripheral horizontal linear shadows 1–2 cm long and 1 mm thick ('Kerley B lines').
- Pleural effusions (usually small and bilateral but can be large and unilateral).
- Peri-hilar shadowing ('batwing' shadowing). Implies acute severe oedema.
- Peri-bronchial cuffing (wall thickening of large proximal airways).
- Multiple ill-defined nodules (air-space shadowing) seen bilaterally (late severe sign).
- Widespread consolidative pattern with air bronchograms. Can be indistinguishable from diffuse infection.
- Normal CTR seen in ARDS compared with increased CTR in pulmonary oedema.

Common pitfalls

Signs of pulmonary oedema are usually bilateral, but can be unilateral, e.g. ITU patient nursed on their side, unilateral aspiration or re-expansion pulmonary oedema after treatment of large pleural effusion.

COPD and asthma

The CXR of patients with chronic airway obstruction often displays features of lung hyperinflation with no focal abnormality.

CXR features of chronic airway obstruction

- Lung hyperexpansion, causing flattening of the hemidiaphragms and increased lucency ('black lungs').
- Dome of diaphragm lies below anterior aspect of seventh rib.
- Abrupt tapering of the peripheral vasculature.
- Presence of bullae (much more common in COPD than in asthma). Basal predominance for bullae is highly suggestive of alpha-1-antitrypsin deficiency.
- Enlarged pulmonary arteries or right heart (as a result of chronic hypoxia).

If these background changes are observed, look for the common complications associated with COPD and asthma.

Complications
- PTX and surgical emphysema.
- Pneumomediastinum.
- Infection.
- Malignancy.
- Bronchiectasis (abnormally dilated airways which can contain fluid levels).
- Allergic bronchopulmonary aspergillosis.

Further imaging

Other imaging modalities are rarely needed in the acute setting. The main use of CT in the acute setting would be to identify a pneumothorax on a background of extensive bullous changes.

Massive haemoptysis

Life-threatening haemoptysis requires urgent resuscitation (📖 Chapter 6). The most common causes of massive haemoptysis and the associated CXR features are as follows.

CXR features
- Irregular focal mass: probably lung primary malignancy eroding an adjacent vessel.
- Consolidation: suggests infection. TB possible.
- Cavity and soft tissue mass: aspergilloma.
- Cavity with air–fluid level: lung abscess.
- Well-defined focal mass: arterio-venous malformation (AVM). Look for tubular feeding vessel. Multiple AVMs seen in Osler–Weber–Rendu syndrome.
- Dilated tubular bronchi or multiple cystic lucencies: bronchiectasis of any cause, but especially cystic fibrosis.

Further imaging may be required, usually CT of the thorax with contrast. A bronchial angiogram may be required when embolization can also be performed as a therapeutic procedure. This needs to be performed at a specialist centre.

Lobar collapse

Lobar collapse (also known as 'atelectasis') is easy to miss on the frontal CXR unless it is specifically looked for. In the elderly patient an underlying malignancy is by far the most common cause, whereas an inhaled foreign body or mucus plug are more likely aetiologies in young patients. Whatever the cause, it is not a diagnosis that can be missed without consequence for the patient. Identifying the affected lobe will guide subsequent investigations, especially bronchoscopy.

General features of lobar collapse

- Opacification of the lobe.
- Displacement of the fissures (especially the horizontal).
- Volume loss on the affected side.
- Upward or downward shift of the hilum towards the collapsed lobe.
- Mediastinal shift towards the side of collapse.
- Poorly defined hemi-diaphragm/mediastinal contours (normally clearly seen).
- Elevation of the hemi-diaphragm.
- Rib crowding (best seen by comparing the gap between ribs on both sides).
- Hyperexpansion of the other lung, causing hyperlucency.
- Complete collapse of the entire lung causes opacification of the whole hemithorax, and ipsilateral shift of the mediastinum and trachea (Fig. 58.10).

Lobar-specific features

Lobar collapse is one of the few indications for performing a lateral CXR if the frontal view is not confirmatory.

- **RLL** Collapses posteriorly and inferiorly. Right hemi-diaphragm obscured.
- **RML** Collapses anteriorly and medially, obscuring right heart border. Triangular opacity on lateral CXR.
- **RUL** Collapses medially and superiorly
- **LUL** (Fig. 58.11) Moves anteriorly and superiorly, creating a 'veil-like' appearance of the left hemi-thorax. Left heart border obscured. A crescent of aerated lung is often seen between the aortic arch and collapsed LUL (hyperexpanded apical segment of LLL).
- **LLL** (Fig. 58.12) The easiest lobar collapse to miss. Collapses posteriorly and inferiorly. Left hemidiaphragm obscured. Can appear as a triangular density behind the heart (the 'sail' sign). Often seen after cardiac surgery.

Further imaging

Post-IV contrast CT of the thorax is the next investigation, either before or after bronchoscopy.

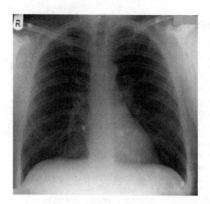

Fig. 58.1 Normal CXR. The heart size is normal and there are no focal lung lesions. Note how the heart borders and hemi-diaphragms are clearly visible.

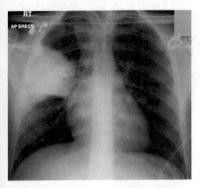

Fig. 58.2 Right upper lobe consolidation. There is abnormal opacity outlining a lung segment. An air bronchogram is seen adjacent to the right hilum.

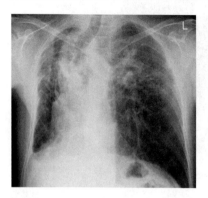

Fig. 58.3 Upper lobe fibrosis. Previous TB infection has caused extensive fibrotic change in the right upper lobe, with volume loss (note the elevated right hilum and tracheal shift), on a background of diffuse reticulonodular shadowing.

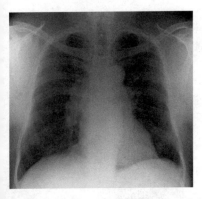

Fig. 58.4 Bilateral hilar lymphadenopathy. The hila are abnormally large and dense in this patient with sarcoid (compare with normal appearance in Fig. 58.1).

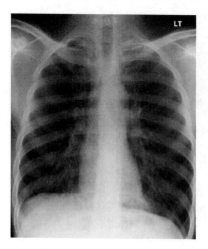

Fig. 58.5 Small pneumothorax. Abnormal lucency is seen parallel to the left lateral chest wall, and a thin vertical line is present (representing the pleural edge). No mediastinal shift has occurred.

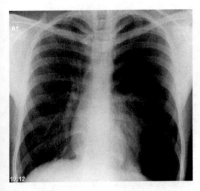

Fig. 58.6 Tension pneumothorax. There is complete collapse of the left lung, extensive air in the left pleural space, and mediastinal shift to the right.

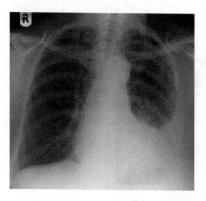

Fig. 58.7 Pleural effusion. Pleural fluid in the left pleural space is seen as abnormal opacity, with a meniscus extending along the lateral chest wall.

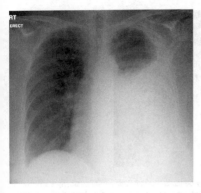

Fig. 58.8 Large pleural effusion. Extensive left-sided pleural fluid, causing shift of the trachea and mediastinum to the right.

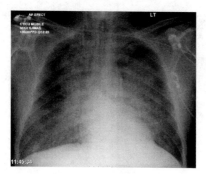

Fig. 58.9 Severe pulmonary oedema. 'Bat-wing', or peri-hilar air-space shadowing. Thin horizontal interstitial lines are seen laterally at the right base (Kerley B lines).

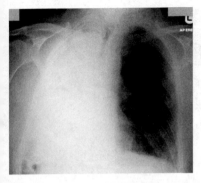

Fig. 58.10 Complete collapse of right lung. A proximal tumour is causing complete collapse of the right lung, seen as a 'white-out' with the trachea shifted *towards* the side of collapse (compare with a large pleural effusion which will shift the mediastinum *away*).

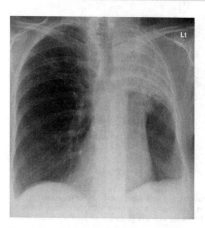

Fig. 58.11 Left upper lobe collapse. There is a mediastinal shift to the left, the left hilum is elevated, and there is abnormal density in the left upper zone. There is marked volume loss in the left hemithorax.

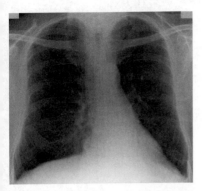

Fig. 58.12 Left lower lobe collapse. The lobe is completely collapsed, and is seen as a dense triangle behind the heart. The left hilum is depressed, the mediastinum has shifted to the left, and the left hemithorax is of reduced volume.

Index